Greta L. Bennett

THE GOD WHO SEES YOU

Devotional Journal for the Family Caregiver

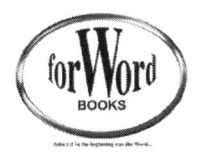

forWord
BOOKS

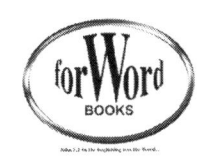

The God Who Sees You
Published by ForWord Books
21143 Hawthorne Blvd, Ste 184
Torrance, CA 90503

Scripture quotations are taken or paraphrased from the following versions of The Holy Bible: American Standard Version (ASV), Christian Standard Bible/Version (CSB/CSV), King James Version (KJV), The Message (MSG), New American Standard Bible/Version (NASB/NASV), New Century Version (NCV), New International Version (NIV), New Living Translation (NLT), New Life Version (NLV), and The Living Bible (TLB).

Lyrics printed of the following hymns are considered Public Domain:

What A Friend We Have in Jesus (UMH 526)
AUTHOR/WORDS: Joseph Medlicott Scriven, 1855
MUSIC: Charles Converse (CONVERSE), 1868

Count Your Blessings
AUTHOR/WORDS: Johnson Oatman, Jr., 1897
MUSIC: Edwin O. Excell, 1897

ISBN 979-8-9882642-3-1

Copyright © 2023 by Greta L. Bennett

All rights reserved. No part of this book may be reproduced or transmitted in any form or by any means, electronic or mechanical, including recording and photocopying, or by any information storage and retrieval system, without written permission from the publisher.

Published in the United States by ForWord Books

DEDICATION

This devotional journal is dedicated to all the family caregivers who have answered God's call to care for one of His precious children. The journey will not be easy, but if you continue to trust God, He will see you through!

PREFACE

The God Who Sees You Devotional Journal for the Family Caregiver is designed to strengthen and encourage you as a family caregiver. You are a part of the 19% of family caregivers who aid an adult with basic medical or functional needs. This is what I did for twelve years, caring for my mother, who had Alzheimer's.

My story as a caregiver began in Hawaii when my then eighty-two-year-old mother came to live with me. Within two years of living with me, she was diagnosed with Alzheimer's, and the roller coaster began. I consider myself a mature Christian, yet her diagnosis shook me. I asked why her, why me, and how this would change my life. Could I still accomplish all the dreams I had? I believe these questions are not unique to me but are something all caregivers ask. This devotional will help you acknowledge your emotions, heal your anxiety, and build a deeper relationship with God, yourself, and your loved one.

The devotional journal is divided into seven sections, each corresponding to an emotion I experienced during my caregiving season. You do not have to go in order; you can choose a section depending on what you are facing that day. If you are a parent who is caring for a child with a disability, grief may not be the section you need; yet I would encourage you to look at a few of the devotionals because you may be grieving for the things that your child will not be able to do. We are caregivers in many ways, but the underlying thing that draws us into community is our love for our loved ones.

I want you to know that I am on this journey with you. The devotional journal is designed to be interactive, with me giving you questions of reflection, action steps, or prayers to recite. You have answered God's call to care for HIS precious child, and your obedience to His call demonstrates your faith in Him. Now, let's get started and see what God has to say to you!

ACKNOWLEDGMENTS

This devotional journal would not have been possible if it were not for the special group of friends God surrounded me with during my season of caregiving.

First, many thanks go out to Rev. Alexis Connor and Deloris Hariston for being my sisters in Hawaii. Both women came alongside me and helped shoulder the burden as I embarked on my caregiving season. They provided much-needed respite, love, and friendship.

Next are Dr. Doris and Dr. Michael Mays. They knew and loved my mother and provided family, friendship, and respite while we lived in Tampa, Florida. They considered my mother their mother and cared for her when I needed a weekend break.

Many thanks go to my publisher, ForWord Books, Larry, Paris, and Langston Rodgers, for bringing my book to fruition. Thank you for believing in me, for holding my hand throughout the publishing process, and for helping to make my dream come true.

Lastly, my heart of gratitude goes out to Deborah Sullivan, who was a caregiver to my mother and me while we lived in Tampa, Florida. The love, compassion, laughter, and care Deborah gave my mother for four years while employed as a caregiver brought tears to my eyes. I know my mother loved her and Deborah, my mother. Although Deborah was our professional caregiver, she quickly became family, and I think of her as an older sister (she did like to boss me around a lot). Her presence allowed me the space and time to craft this journal, for which I am forever grateful, as well as many other acts of kindness she gave.

TABLE OF CONTENTS

INTRODUCTION
viii

CHAPTER ONE
Frustration
1

CHAPTER TWO
Anger
23

CHAPTER THREE
Fear and Worry
53

CHAPTER FOUR
Loneliness
88

CHAPTER FIVE
Tired or Weariness
115

CHAPTER SIX
Sorrow
138

CHAPTER SEVEN
Grief
162

INTRODUCTION

In 2009 my mother came to live with me in my Army assignment in Hawaii. She was 81 years old. What neither of us knew was that three years later, she would be diagnosed with Alzheimer's.

Suddenly I was thrown into the world of care-giving and I was scared. As I embarked on this journey, God used it to show me that I wasn't the "super" Christian I thought I was, but He lovingly held a mirror to let me see what He saw, and it wasn't pretty.

A caregiver is defined by me as a person with whom God has trusted the life support of another. Yes, you, as the caregiver, are a life support to the person whom you are caring for. At times it will be fulfilling but to be honest most of the time it's just hard, but never too hard for those who have put their complete trust in Jesus Christ. His words are full of life support for you, the caregiver.

In this devotional, I will share with you, scriptures that will not only help you make it through your caregiving journey but also to come out of this journey victorious!

The devotional is divided into the emotions I experienced during my caregiving season: Frustration, Anger, Fear and Worry, Loneliness, Tired or Weariness, Sorrow and Grief.

Each emotional section has a daily scripture, devotion, and space for you to journal your thoughts based on guided questions and suggestions. This book is to be your chronicle. In the end, you will be able to look back and see how far you have grown in your relationship with yourself, your loved ones, and God.

Know that God is no respecter of persons; what He did for me, He WILL DO FOR YOU; just TRUST HIM!

CHAPTER ONE
Frustration

One of the emotions you will encounter frequently will be frustration. It comes from expectations, and you can become frustrated when things do not go as planned. Having expectations is not wrong; however, ensuring that your expectations are not unrealistic will be wise. My biggest frustration stemmed from the healthcare system. Trying to arrange the appropriate care and medications and working with several healthcare providers who did not talk to each other...FRUSTRATION!

Sometimes I got frustrated with my mother for her stubbornness in not adhering to what I had planned and then at myself for noting being as "on it" as I thought I should be. You see how expectations are the fuel for frustration. Once again, there's nothing wrong with having expectations, but it is probably wise to build with the expectation that not all things will work out as you have planned.

FEELING UNDERDRESSED

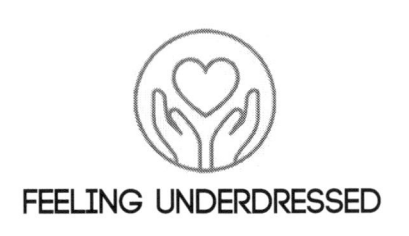

"Finally, be strong in the Lord and in his mighty power. Put on the full armor of God, so that you can take your stand against the devil's schemes." Ephesians 6:10-11 (NIV)

We wear clothes to protect our precious and sensitive skin from the elements. Our skin, in turn, protects our insides. We as Christians also have a "dress code" we are to have when we "go outside," and that is the armor of God. And that armor does the same thing as our clothes and skin, which protects us from the outside world, providing a protective barrier between our souls and the enemy.

Often when we feel overwhelmed or stressed, it's because we are naked and therefore experiencing the full brunt of Satan's attacks! Now if that picture doesn't frighten you, it should. How can you defeat the enemy without being properly dressed? You can't! The responsibility is yours to ensure that you dress for battle every day! The days will be filled with minor attacks, some not so much, but if you have the full armor of God, you can withstand the enemy. So, Get Dressed!

ACTION STEPS:

- Read Ephesians 6:14-18, and consciously say out loud: Today I put on my helmet of salvation. I, therefore, am mindful that I am saved, and my actions reflect God. I put on my belt of truth and will be truthful in all my actions. I put on my vest of righteousness, being in right standing with God because of the blood of Jesus. I put on my shoes of peace. I do not cause chaos or disputes but bring peace to all situations. I carry my faith like a shield to remind me that I have a Savior who has made way for me, and because He lives, I do. And finally, I will surrender to the Holy Spirit within me to actively remember the word of God and use it to protect me against the ideas the enemy may put in my thoughts or any obstacle he may place in my path. I will start and end each day with thanksgiving and prayer to the Lord.

ARE YOU WEARY

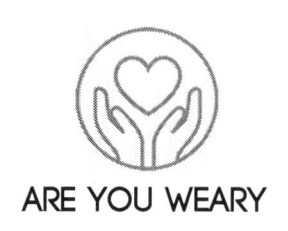

"Come to me, all of you who are weary and burdened, and I will give you rest. Take up my yoke and learn from me, because I am lowly and humble in heart, and you will find rest for your souls. For my yoke is easy and my burden is light."
Matthew 11:28-30 (CSV)

Caring for someone can be extremely exhausting! You are the go-to person for EVERYTHING. The question is, to whom do you go to get refreshed and exhale? The answer is Jesus. He is the very first person whom you should run to for help. He tells us to come to Him, He knows that this world is hard, and the demands can sometimes be unreasonable. Each day you are bombarded with a different scenario where you must decide. Oh, how you long for a routine, but you get chaos and more bad news instead. This is the time to STOP and run to Jesus, tell Him about your struggles, and give Him the authority to help you. See, He is there waiting for YOU to come to Him and ask. So today, make the decision not to do it all alone. Give it to Jesus, and let Him carry you.

REFLECTIONS:

- Do you feel as if you are alone and have no one to help?
- Have you been trying to do everything on your own?
- Can you prioritize the daily demands and get assistance with those things that you don't have to do yourself?

ACTION STEPS:

- List those things YOU must do and those you can seek help for.
- Once the list is completed, research to find someone to help you. Feel free to seek professional caregivers or government assistance; ask for the help you need!

PRAYER:

Dear Lord, I confess my need to give all this to You. I can't handle it alone; frankly, I don't want to handle it alone. Please help me. I ask that You open doors of assistance to me. Give me wisdom and discernment to choose between the services needed and the person to assist. And above all, help me to make You a priority in my life, not just during this season but for a lifetime, in Jesus' Name, Amen.

IT'S JUST TOO MUCH

> "We demolish arguments and every pretension that sets itself up against the knowledge of God, and we take captive every thought to make it obedient to Christ." 2 Corinthians 10:5 (NIV)

Have you had those days when you just wanted to scream? I mean, scream and then walk away from the responsibilities and all the demands that are being placed on you? I did. I found that when I wanted to leave, it was because I had begun to listen to the voices in my head that told me caregiving was too hard, that I deserved better, that I would lose myself, and on and on. Looking closely, you will see that I was focused on myself, not my mother but me. I allowed the enemy to change my focus from God and my mother to poor little me! But once I made up my mind and decided that I was going to speak to the truth of who I was in Christ, the voices went away, and I began to see things a lot clearer. The idea of my being a caregiver for my mother didn't scare me or overwhelm me. I was no longer frustrated with the new life I had to live as a caregiver.

Today's scripture challenges you to stop listening to all the voices that are telling you that you are ill-equipped for this journey; the voice that pulls you from looking at God to looking at you; the voices of all the people who are there to help but are just adding more confusion. STOP and take all those voices to God and allow Him to filter what and whom you should listen too.

ACTION STEPS:

- Find your quiet place and take a notepad and pencil.
- Write down all thoughts (thoughts of feeling inadequate, lonely, unsure, etc.) you wish to give to God…Hint it should be all of them.
- After writing them down, have a long conversation with your Savior and ask Him to bring clarity and discernment.

HEAR MY CRY

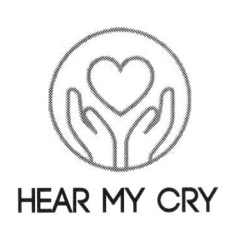

"God, hear my cry; pay attention to my prayer. I call to you from the ends of the earth when my heart is without strength. Lead me to a rock that is high above me, for you have been a refuge for me, a strong tower in the face of the enemy. I will dwell in your tent forever and take refuge under the shelter of your wings."
Psalm 61:1-4 (CSB)

God hears you! He is paying attention to your prayers. The more challenging question is, are you listening to His answers? As you pour your heart out to the Lord, weak from the burden of caring for your loved one and unable to see any way forward, that is when you are in the best position to hear from God. He is your strong tower, and you are to run to Him. You will find comfort, strength, and answers to your prayers in Him.

Yes, dear one, He hears you!

REFLECTIONS:

- What does a place of refuge bring to your mind?
- Do you visualize that place you have just described in God?
- Identify what you can do to help you see God as a place of refuge.
- Engage in a conversation with your heavenly Father.

FINDING PEACE THROUGH THE CHAOS

"Don't worry about anything, but in everything, through prayer and petition with thanksgiving, present your request to God. And the peace of God, which surpasses all understanding, will guard your hearts and minds in Christ Jesus." Philippians 4:6-7 (CSV)

You have a million things to do now as if you didn't have a million before this season of caring for your loved one. You just got more on your plate. A plate I'm sure you thought was pretty full already. In this situation, God knows you CAN handle a little more. Remember, He is still in control, and this season only caught you by surprise, not Him. The fact that this is now added to your plate means YOU CAN HANDLE this...with Christ. Christ is your secret weapon! Having a relationship with Him also allows you to bring EVERYTHING to Him. You are to seek his guidance, ask for help and lay everything at His feet. Today's scripture reinforces this. Once you bring EVERYTHING to Him, and by EVERYTHING, I mean everything, the hurt, the anger, the worry, the frustration, whatever you are experiencing today, Jesus wants to handle it FOR YOU!! Once you unload, then allow His peace to comfort you, and although there is chaos, you will experience a peace that even you can't explain.

REFLECTIONS:

- Do you know that you can tell Jesus anything?
- Are you ready to unload your cares for today?
- Ask Jesus for help today.
- Share your concerns with Him.

LEARNING TO BE SILENT

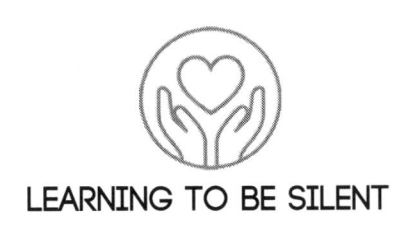

> "But Moses said to the people, 'Don't be afraid. Stand firm and see the Lord's salvation that he will accomplish for you today; for the Egyptians you see today, you will never see again. The Lord will fight for you, and you must be quiet.'"
> Exodus 14:13-14 (CSV)

You are not in this alone! I know the enemy wants you to believe you are, but you are not. Your God is fighting for you and has everything already worked out for your good and the good of your loved one. Often, we see the enemy coming. The enemy is the form of bills, relationships that aren't working well, car breaking down, bad news, illnesses, etc. But just as Moses reminded the Israelites, I remind you to STAND FIRM and know that God is fighting for you. Your role is to continue to place your trust in Him while remaining silent.

Being silent for today's lesson means not speaking about the negativity around you, not focusing on all that is going "wrong," and not confronting an issue or person out of anger or bitterness. Instead, speak words of life and reflect on all the good things God has done for you while reminding yourself of who you are: YOU are a son or daughter of the MOST HIGH God! A God who loves you fights for you and has already made way for you to defeat the enemies today!

ACTION STEPS:

- List all the "enemies" you have today, any issue that has you afraid of tomorrow or that is worrying you.
- Now, turn this list into a prayer request to the Lord and then be silent.

HEARING DESPITE THE NOISE

> "When my spirit was overwhelmed within me,
> You knew my path. In the way where I walk
> They have hidden a trap for me." Psalm 142:3 (NASB)

Learning to hear God amid all the chaos is the secret to overcoming versus being overwhelmed. On any given day, you can face so many decisions: should you change doctors, which healthcare plan is right, does the house need to be renovated to accommodate the needs of your loved one, and on and on they come. Yet, the answers will come if you have spent time with God and allowed Him to minister to your soul. The contrast is diving headfirst and making decisions without God's counsel. The first brings peace, the latter chaos and frustration.

In this season, more than ever, you need God; you need Him to help YOU while you help your loved one. While there are "hidden traps" by the enemy, keeping close fellowship with God will expose them and reduce their impact so you may continue the path God has directed. Remember, He has enlisted you to care for His son or daughter, and as you grow in your relationship with God, you will see that your caregiving is a loving response to God for His love toward you.

REFLECTIONS:

- Do I really hear God?
- Have I allowed myself to cultivate a relationship with Him in His word?
- Are there things that I can do to foster a more intimate relationship with God?
- Talk with your heavenly Father.

REDIRECT YOUR MIND

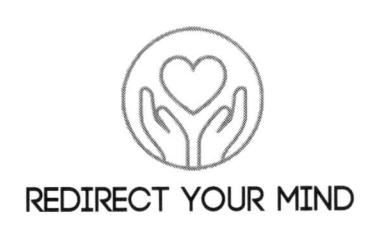

> "Finally, brothers and sisters, whatever is true, whatever is noble, whatever is right, whatever is pure, whatever is lovely, whatever is admirable—if anything is excellent or praiseworthy—think about such things." Philippians 4:8 (NIV)

Sometimes when the world around you is too much, and the noise overwhelms you, it's time to think about something pleasant. I know that sounds trite, but that's exactly what Paul is telling the believers in Philippi. Think about what you know about God! Reflect on how good He has been to you; remember how He has been there for you throughout your lifetime. In other words, redirect your thoughts from the current and think about God! His word says He is the same yesterday, today, and tomorrow. He does not change what He did for you a year ago; know that He will do it again today!

Once you begin to reflect on God, today is put into its proper place... in the hands of God versus in your head! Yes, you will have decisions, chores, and errands, BUT remembering the goodness of God will keep you from feeling overwhelmed and remind you how unbelievably loved you are!

REFLECTIONS:

Remember this hymn?

"Count Your Blessings"

When upon life's billows you are tempest-tossed,
When you are discouraged, thinking all is lost,
Count your many blessings; name them one by one,
And it will surprise you what the Lord has done.

(Chorus)
Count your blessings;
Name them one by one.
Count your blessings;
See what God hath done.

Are you ever burdened with a load of care?
Does the cross seem heavy you are called to bear?
Count your many blessings; ev'ry doubt will fly,
And you will be singing as the days go by.

(Chorus)

When you look at others with their lands and gold,
Think that Christ has promised you his wealth untold.
Count your many blessings; money cannot buy
Your reward in heaven nor your home on high.

(Chorus)

So, amid the conflict, whether great or small,
Do not be discouraged; God is over all.
Count your many blessings; angels will attend,
Help and comfort give you to your journey's end.

(Chorus)

DON'T SWEAT THE SMALL STUFF

"A soldier on duty doesn't get caught up in making deals at the marketplace. He concentrates on carrying out orders. An athlete who refuses to play by the rules will never get anywhere. It's the diligent farmer who gets the produce. Think it over. God will make it all plain." 2 Timothy 2:4-7 (The Message)

Learning to prioritize is crucial as a caregiver. Of all the demands that will come to you, you must discern what must be done now and what can wait for tomorrow and identify what doesn't need to be done! Our scripture teaches just that: to know your tasks and focus on them, not looking to the left or the right but straight ahead at the path God has laid out for you.

As you determine what must be done, then set your mind on them and get to it. There may be times when you have to adjust your plans because something unexpected that has to be done that day comes up, then you adjust. But you must make your plan and work toward that plan every day. You will see what you have accomplished at the end of the day!

ACTION STEPS:

- Get a notepad and title it Your To-Do List.
- Each day write out what must be done.
- At each entry put, draw a square box. As you complete each task, shade the box, that way, a glance at your list will let you know what has been achieved and what has not. However, if you could only complete a portion of it, then only color half of the box.
- At the end of the day, when you review your list, you will see what was accomplished and what wasn't.

DO YOU TRUST GOD

> "Jesus looked hard at them and said, 'No chance at all if you think you can pull it off yourself. Every chance in the world if you trust God to do it.'" Matthew 19:26 (The Message)

Your caregiving journey will be an exciting one... once you learn whom you can trust. Initially, it will be hard and difficult, but it will get easier as you turn to God and really and truly trust Him with everything. Easier in the sense that you will realize that God is really in control, and you really need and want Him to be! It will not get easier emotionally; the person you care for may not get any better, and watching them advance or succumb to the disease will tear you apart. No, that will never get easier; however, as you trust God and you see Him actively working in your situation, you will have peace within you. You'll learn not to get all worked up over that particular day's issues but to put it in God's hands and patiently wait for Him to instruct you in what you must do for His plan to come to fruition.

Your God loves you and your loved one, and although you may not understand why this particular season, you will know that you are better in His care than without. Yes, with God, you can and will overcome this!

REFLECTIONS:

- Have you been trying to do things yourself, or perhaps you are like me and go to God for help but then "help" Him with suggestions?
- Take time to reflect on how much of your life and yourself you've truly turned over to God.
- Talk with your heavenly Father (tell Him how you feel and what you need help with).

WHERE IS YOUR TRUST

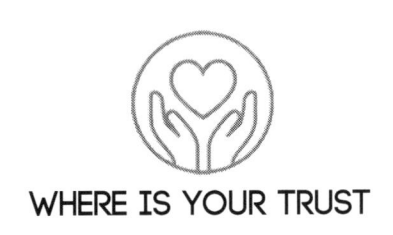

"Trust in the Lord with all your heart, and do not rely on your own understanding; in all your ways know him, and he will make your paths straight." Proverbs 3:5-6 (CSV)

What is your relationship with Christ? Have you accepted Him as your Savior? Do you know Him as a friend? It is a latter position (friend) where you begin to grow in knowing Him. Think about some of the good friends that you have. What do you do to cultivate that relationship? Do you call them often and catch up on the events in their lives? Do you schedule outings to hang out and physically see each other? Do you think of them often and sometimes send them a little gift? All of these things that you do with your earthly friends, God expects and wants that from you. Spending time with Him and "catching up" is prayer, going for a walk or a lunch where you and Jesus commune together, you feel His presence, and you know He's there. And the gifts you bring Him are your time, attention, trust, and obedience to Him. Do you spend time with your friend Jesus? Does He know everything that's going on with you? Do you hear His soft voice instructing you in your next steps?

See, as you chat with Jesus, you become familiar with how He speaks with you through the Holy Spirit. When you hear the voice of the Spirit, do EXACTLY as He instructs. Putting your trust in Jesus is never wrong; it is the absolute best and the only thing you, as His child, should do.

REFLECTIONS:

- Do you trust God?
- How are you trusting God?
- Is it evident in your daily life?
- Are there areas in which you can trust Him more?
- Talk with your heavenly Father.

KNOW WHAT'S IN THE ENEMY'S ARSENAL

"'...no weapon forged against you will prevail, and you will refute every tongue that accuses you. This is the heritage of the servants of the Lord, and this is their vindication from me,' declares the Lord." Isaiah 54:17 (NIV)

You do know you have a target on your back, right? It was placed there the moment you accepted Christ as your Savior. Yes, the enemy put a giant bullseye on your back and is determined to steal, kill and destroy you. His attacks can be horrific but often more subtle, and one weapon he uses is confusion and chaos!

All the demands that are being placed on you now...some may be the enemy trying to distract you from your purpose. What is your purpose? It is to trust God, to provide the best care you can for your loved one, and again to trust God. Remember, your God gives you His peace, a sign that you are walking in His will is peace which contrasts with what the enemy does, which is to bring noise and confusion. However, you being a child of the Most High God means that whatever weapon the enemy attempts to use on you will not work. Turn your attention away from the noise and focus on God!

ACTION STEPS:
- Read today's scripture out loud and remember that NO weapon formed against YOU will prosper throughout the day!

YOU CAN HANDLE MORE THAN YOU THINK

> "…but those who trust in the Lord will renew their strength; they will soar on wings like eagles; they will run and not become weary, they will walk and not faint." Isaiah 40:31 (CSV)

This scripture, if rephrased, would be, "You are made to handle more than you think." See, you are God's design, He is the architect, and He knows exactly how much weight you can bear. I know I have said this before, but it's worth repeating. The fact that you are going through this journey proves you can handle it. God never gives you more than you can handle, and today's scripture shows why. Once you put your complete trust in Him, He takes over and becomes your strength. It's as if you have been given superhuman strength to handle this journey. You are infused with God!!!

Now that you have been infused with God's strength, do the challenges of today stand any chance of defeating you? I think not.

ACTION STEPS:

- Being overwhelmed or frustrated is something all caregivers go through, yet you know now that you can handle this journey. Today, look in the mirror and see yourself as capable, strong, and loved by God. Then say to yourself:

    "I can tackle the challenges for today because God is with me."

    "I am strong in the Lord."

    "God loves me."

DON'T GIVE UP

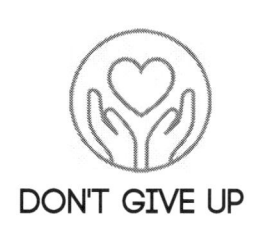

"Let us not get tired of doing good, for we will reap at the proper time if we don't give up." Galatians 6:9 (CSV)

I'm sure there are days when you want to throw in the towel, grab your keys, get in the car, and drive away!!! But what stops you? Is it that you love the person whom you are caring for? Could it be that you know this season is directly tied to God's will for you? Remember, nothing happens by chance for those who believe in Jesus. He uses all aspects of life to mold us and shape us into His image. I want you to know that this season is as much about you as it is about the person you care for. So please don't give up, don't give up on them, and don't give up on yourself. Continue to trust God and know that this season will pass, and you and your loved one will be better for it, whatever the outcome.

REFLECTIONS:

- How do you view your role as a caregiver?
- Is it something you have embraced, or are you fighting the new role?
- You may ask, "What can I do to help alleviate some of the load of caregiving?"
- Get someone to come and sit for a couple of hours, join a support group, etc.
- Talk with your heavenly Father.

REFLECTIONS
ACTION STEPS
PRAYERS

CHAPTER TWO

Anger

Don't let anyone tell you that you don't have the right to be angry because YOU DO. It is a natural response to a drastic, unexpected, and immediate change in your life. Having the responsibility of being a person's sole provider is hard. Most of us do not plan for a scenario such as this, where all of your plans are now placed on the back burner, if not canceled in their entirety, because of the needs of another. Sometimes this person is a person whom you love; still, you have the right to be angry. Sometimes, it is caring for a person who has not shown appreciation for you or the relationship; yes, you have the right to be angry. However, regardless of which scenario you find yourself in, whether you love the person or not, whether you like the person or not, whether the person recognizes you or not, whether the person never apologizes for the things they said or did…you do not have the right to be angry forever. It is the releasing of the anger that you free yourself (Ephesians 4:26 NLT, "And 'don't sin by letting anger control you.' Don't let the sun go down while you are still angry,").

The scriptures that follow are here to remind you of WHOSE you are and Who you are as a daughter or son of the Most High God. There will be many scriptures taken from Proverbs that reinforce how being angry isn't the best course of action, and there will be scriptures from the New Testament on anger. All are designed to help you understand yourself as God's child.

WHAT'S IN YOUR HEART

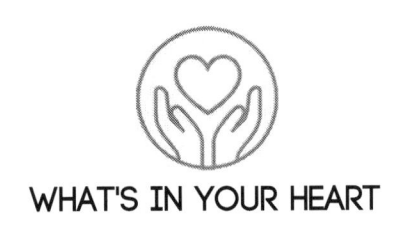

"You shall not hate your fellow countryman in your hearts; you may surely reprove your neighbor, but shall not incur sin because of him. You shall not take vengeance, nor bear any grudge against the sons of your people, but you shall love your neighbor as yourself; I am the Lord." Leviticus 19:17-18 (NASV)

Your heart is fertile ground; therefore, be careful what you put into it because it WILL grow. As you begin to settle into your role as caregiver, it can be easy to blame others for the situation, you can blame the person you are caring for, and you can blame yourself; however, is that what God wants for you? The scripture above suggests it is not. God has no tolerance for a heart full of anger, hate, and blame and one that holds grudges. Why? Because you stop looking toward the Lord to meet your needs, you can no longer see the blessing daily because you are consumed with hate, judgment, and envy. Your Lord wants YOUR total attention! He has demonstrated what is in His heart, LOVE, and He wants the same for you. Even though you have heard this several times over, release the hurt and anger you are carrying and allow God's love to guide you toward becoming a more loving caregiver and individual.

REFLECTIONS:

- Do you have something to release to the Lord?
- How can you demonstrate your Love for the Lord through your caregiving?
- Confess anything in your heart hindering you from fully submitting to your role as a caregiver.
- Talk with your heavenly Father.

CONFESS

"What is the source of quarrels and conflicts among you? Is not the source your pleasures that wage war in your members? You lust and do not have; so you commit murder. You are envious and cannot obtain; so you fight and quarrel. You do not have because you do not ask." James 4:1-2 (NASV)

James cuts to the heart of the issues with our anger...it's US! We want what we do not have, and that "lack" festers into an open wound of hurt, yet it manifests itself as anger, disconnection, and envy. Do not be fooled in this season of caregiving. It can be really tempting to look to others whose grass appears to be greener but do not buy into it. Everyone will have or has had their fair share of heartache and trials and tribulations; Jesus Himself tells us so. Yet, Jesus reinforces that we are to take courage in Him because He has overcome the world.

Right now, your world may look bleak, restricted, and hopeless. BUT it is not. Do not allow your perception of "lack" within your life to bring you to an area of envy and anger that causes you to lash out at others. ASK God to heal your anger and hurt. ASK Him to help you release the anxiety that is in your heart; then, once you have asked, release and allow Him to work in your heart, your attitude, life, and situation.

REFLECTIONS:

- Am I unhappy? Why or why not?
- Have I longed for someone else's life?
- Has my attitude caused me to be unkind to others?
- Is it difficult to accept the season I am in?
- Talk to your heavenly Father.

GETTING TO THE HEART OF THE MATTER

"He who is slow to anger has great understanding, but he who is quick-tempered exalts folly." Proverbs 14:29 (NASV)

We've now examined several scriptures instructing us to be slow to anger, right? Why would the Lord see fit to put this into scripture so many times? Because we are a thick-headed people and we need to be told several times and in several different ways. In looking at this scripture, we see that by being able to control one's temper, we actually allow ourselves to see the bigger picture and gain a healthier perspective of our loved one, the disease/illness, and us.

Anger gets in the way of us really seeing the situation and inhibits us from looking at it from a godly perspective. YOU are a child of God, and as His child, you are to seek His counsel and learn to look at your life through His lens. You remember that popular term used in the 90s, "What would Jesus do?" If you use that mindset when it comes to this season, your focus shifts to God versus you, and you begin to receive His understanding of what He wants YOU to do in this season. Learn to let go and then listen for His voice.

REFLECTIONS:

- Can I let my anger go?
- Is my anger interfering with my relationship with God?
- Talk with your heavenly Father.

ARE YOU A HOT HEAD

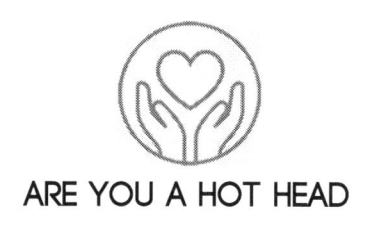

> "A hot-tempered man stirs up strife, but the slow to anger calms a dispute." Proverbs 15:18 (NASV)

Let's do some self-reflecting. Are you quick to get angry? Is it easier for you to see what needs to be corrected versus what is good? Are you a glass-half-empty person? Do little things, when not done correctly, really get your goat? Then, my friend, you may be classified as hot-headed. While there isn't anything wrong with being a critical thinker or a person who can see the potential pitfalls in ideas, there must be a balance. You are in a season that may last for some time, and being quick-tempered will only add unnecessary stress to an already stressful situation. It is time to see the glass half full now. You and the person you are caring for need to have as many positive influences as possible. Surround yourself with positive people, uplifting material, and learn to let go of your temper. Yes, there will be things that will send you through the roof; just ensure that those things are fewer than the things that make you smile.

Put your trust in the Lord and learn to cast all your cares on Him, for He does care for you!

REFLECTIONS:

- Am I hot-tempered?
- Is there room for improvement in my attitude and language?
- How can I begin to be more peaceful?
- Am I creating an atmosphere of peace and positivity?
- Talk to your heavenly Father.

ARE YOU DEFILED

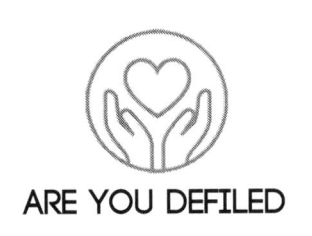

"And He was saying, 'That which proceeds out of the man, that is what defiles the man. For from within, out of the heart of men, proceed the evil thoughts, fornications, thefts, murders, adulteries, deeds of coveting and wickedness, as well as deceit, sensuality, envy, slander pride, and foolishness. All these evil things proceed from within and defile the man.'"
Mark 7:20-23 (NASV)

Wow, I know you're thinking, "That is not me!" but let's look deeper into Jesus' words. Your words and actions are an indicator of what is in your heart! Jesus is forcing us to look at our behavior. There was a school of thought that one's behavior was the root of the source of evil. Jesus contradicts that. It is what is ALREADY in the heart that comes out in our behavior. Many good, God-fearing Christians still exhibit "signs" of an impure heart. The words that come out of their mouth do not bring glory to God but tear others down. Their words do not speak of kindness and compassion but of envy, lies, and gossip. What do the words that come out of your mouth reveal about you?

As a caregiver, YOU are the authority now in the home. Are you honoring God with your words and actions? Is your heart defiled?

REFLECTIONS:

- Look at your behavior; what is it conveying about you?
- Talk with your heavenly Father.

ARE YOU HARBORING HATRED

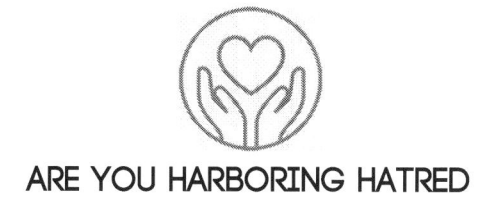

> "Hatred stirs up strife, but love covers all transgressions."
> Proverbs 10:12 (NASV)

Can I ask you a personal question? Are you harboring hate toward your loved one for "putting" you in this situation? If the answer is yes, today's scripture will speak directly to you.

In this life, we will have trials and tribulations. Jesus told us so in John 16:33. None of us will exit this life without "something" throwing us a serious curve ball. Blaming your loved one isn't the answer nor is continuing to blame yourself. In fact, it only makes the situation worse. This may be hard to hear but we know that our lives are in God's hands. Therefore, for His own reasons, He has allowed this season in your lives (you and your loved one) and the question to ask isn't so much as why but what. What will this season teach or produce in you that you wouldn't have without it? God will NEVER give us more than we can handle; His word assures us of this. So first and foremost, you can handle this situation. Two, there is something for you to learn in this situation, and three, this situation can bring you into a closer relationship with God...IF you let it!

REFLECTIONS:

- Am I harboring hate toward my loved one?
- Can I trust God enough to release this hatred to Him?
- Talk with your heavenly Father.

DON'T LET YOUR ANGER GET THE BEST OF YOU

"Cease from anger and forsake wrath; do not fret; it leads only to evildoing." Psalm 37:8 (NASV)

Why is it so important to control your anger? This scripture tells us that it only leads to evildoing. Translation, nothing good comes out of it. When you harbor anger and continue to worry over a situation that perhaps you cannot change, nothing good comes out of it. You begin to fixate on the problem versus focusing on God. You then only see the situation versus seeing the goodness of God IN the situation. You misplace your anger on the individual versus taking it to the Lord, who will help you release it. Being a child of God, you can now take all your cares, hurts, and anger to the Lord. With a humble heart, confess your anger and allow Him to transform you. It's a choice. Which will you choose?

REFLECTIONS:

- Am I worrying about this situation?
- Have I turned all my cares over to the Lord?
- Talk with your heavenly Father.

LOSING YOUR COOL

"A fool always loses his temper, but a wise man holds it back."
Proverbs 29:11 (NASV)

As you establish your "new normal," there will be days when you want to lose your cool. You may want to lash out at your loved one or whoever is close to you…but remember you are no fool; YOU are wise! As children of God, we are to conduct ourselves in a manner that brings God glory in everything we do, including and especially this season of caregiving. Know that you bring honor to the Lord as you care for your loved one. Now that's not to say there won't be days when you slip. Slipping is permissible. Just don't let it be the norm.

REFLECTIONS:
- Do I have triggers that cause me to lose my cool?
- How can I avoid them or at least minimize their effect on me?
- Talk to your heavenly Father.

PUTTING AWAY BITTERNESS

"Let all bitterness and wrath and anger and clamor and slander be put away from you, along with all malice. Be kind to one another, tender-hearted, forgiving each other, just as God in Christ also has forgiven you." Ephesians 4:31-32 (NASV)

Bitterness about your situation can erode your heart and relationships with others and God. Paul instructs the believers in Ephesus to choose to be kind and act lovingly toward each other. You, too, have a choice to be kind. Although, for the moment, you may receive some gratification from "speaking your mind" or being unkind. In the long run, what does it say about YOUR relationship with God?

Remember, it's always about God and your relationship with Him. He allows us to experience hardships and use them as tools to understand better who He is and who we are in relationship to Him. This season isn't just about your loved one or you. It is about YOUR relationship with God and how you allow Him to work within your heart to change your behavior and attitude to align with His.

REFLECTIONS:

- How is my relationship with God?
- Do I read His word and allow it to change me?
- Am I the same person now as I was a year ago?
- Talk to your heavenly Father.

AVOIDING THE TRIGGERS

> "A gentle answer turns away wrath, but a harsh word stirs up anger. The tongue of the wise makes knowledge acceptable, but the mouth of fools spouts folly." Proverbs 15:1-2 (NASV)

As you navigate these waters of caregiving, you will soon figure out what triggers you toward anger. Often times it can be from the very person you are taking care of! Their words can be harsh, ungrateful, unkind, unforgiving, and the list can go on and on, BUT you cannot allow the words or the situation to get the best of you. When your loved one is unkind, reflect on the days when they were kind to you or reflect on a time when you were peaceful and happy. Think about something you have planned to do soon (take a bubble bath, eat some pizza) or anything that will allow you not to respond in kind. How you respond also sends a message to your loved one that YOU are in control and have chosen to be positive and not give in to negativity. Over time, this practice of choosing to be positive will become second nature to you, and you will discover that you have so much to be thankful for, which will be that you have mastered things that trigger you to anger!

REFLECTIONS:

- What are the triggers that spur me toward anger?
- How can I deflect or avoid them?
- Be determined to practice choosing to be positive and record your progress.
- Talk with your heavenly Father.

LEARNING A NEW WAY OF SPEAKING

> "But now you also, put them all aside: anger, wrath, malice, slander, and abusive speech from your mouth."
> Colossians 3:8 (NASV)

Learning to speak peace, love, and kindness can be challenging when you are used to "speaking your mind." As we now know, this isn't helpful to you or your loved one because it does not bring God honor. Yes, that's right, all that we do in this life is to bring honor and glory to God. Look at the words you speak and how you use them when you say them. Does it bring God glory? Dear one, now is the time to learn a new way of speaking. Speak love into your atmosphere; remember, God has given YOU the power to do so. This does not mean that you lie about how you feel. At first, maybe remain silent about your feelings if it will not bring peace or honor. As you learn to be silent, the Spirit of God will show you how to transform your angry words into words that still speak your truth, but it is done so in a way that does not place others on the defensive. It allows them to hear you versus them hearing your emotion. Speaking words of love does not mean saying I love you all the time. It means being mindful of how the words you speak are received and the impact your words have. Learning a new way of speaking is being mindful and respectful of your God, yourself, and others.

REFLECTIONS:

- Are my words harsh and unkind?
- How can I practice speaking words of kindness and love?
- Do my words honor God?
- Talk with your heavenly Father.

MANAGING YOUR ANGER

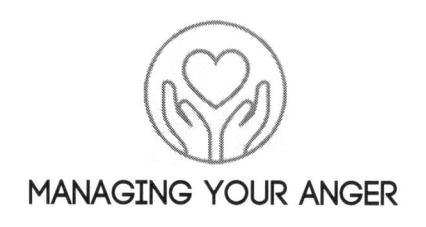

"Be angry, and yet do not sin; do not let the sun go down on your anger, and do not give the devil an opportunity. He who steals must steal no longer; but rather he must labor, performing with his own hands what is good, so that he will have something to share with one who has need. Let no unwholesome word proceed from your mouth, but only such a word as is good for edification according to the need of the moment, so that it will give grace to those who hear. Do not grieve the Holy Spirit of God, by whom you were sealed for the day of redemption. Let all bitterness and wrath and anger and clamor and slander be put away from you, along with all malice. Be kind to one another, tender-hearted, forgiving each other, just as God in Christ also has forgiven you."
Ephesians 4:26-32 (NASV)

This scripture packs a punch! Here we have the apostle Paul instructing the church at Ephesus to not be angry with one another. The assumption is obvious; there was anger amongst the believers. Yet it acknowledges that we do and can get angry at things, circumstances, and each other, but the key is to address it and then LET IT GO! This scripture shows that allowing the anger to fester within our hearts gives room for the devil. And we know that when we allow the devil any access to our lives, he causes chaos and destruction. While Paul is not specific in how the church at Ephesus was sinning, we can assume it was in the form of gossip, lies, and holding grudges, which some could consider minor, but if gestured can cause division, hence why Paul stresses them to be unified in Christ. Therefore, Paul instructs them and us to stop the sin amongst us, which steals our joy individually and collectively and mires our witness for Christ.

Dear one, in this season of caregiving, you may be angry, but now it is time to let it go. Isn't it better to be obedient to the word of God and surrender your anger to Him than to allow it to fester? Allow Him to bring peace to your heart and forgive. I know that is a HUGE word, but forgiving the individual who has harmed you does not mean that you are saying that it was OK for them to do what they did. It means you are no longer allowing it to harm you! The stress and anxiety that it causes you can also manifest physically in the forms of high blood pressure, a stroke, weight gain, or weight loss. Forgiveness releases you from the hold of that hurt, allowing God to work. Allow God to work in you today and ask for His help in you forgiving others so that your anger does not cause you to sin.

REFLECTIONS:

- Why am I angry?
- Do I allow my anger to inhibit me from doing what God has called me to do?
- Has my anger affected my relationships with others?
- Talk to your heavenly Father.
- Write out a letter or prayer to the Lord and express your feelings, asking Him for healing and the ability to be obedient to His word.

TAKE CONTROL OF YOUR ANGER

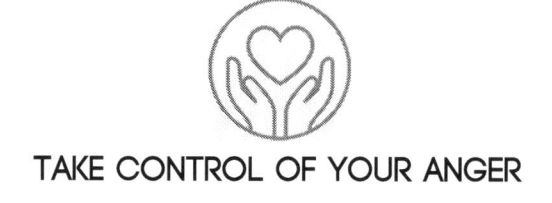

"Do not be eager in your heart to be angry, for anger resides in the bosom of fools." Ecclesiastes 7:9 (NASV)

You have the power to control your thoughts and words, whether you are angry or not. You have the power to CHOOSE to be whatever you wish. In this season, when so much is required of you, is it not better to choose to be peaceful? You lose when you allow your anger to control you, especially over a situation you cannot change. Again, you lose the ability to see your circumstance from a godly perspective; you lose the ability to see the beauty in your loved one and this season of caregiving, and you forfeit your ability to choose!

Once again, we see that choosing to be angry is for unwise and foolish individuals. You can be angry but lose when you allow anger to consume you, and you become foolish. Would you rather be wise or a fool? The choice is yours.

This is the Day that the Lord has made. WILL you rejoice and be glad in it?

REFLECTIONS:

- How often do you choose to be wise?
- Today, reside to be wise in everything you do today.
- Talk with your heavenly Father.

OUR EXAMPLE IS THE LORD

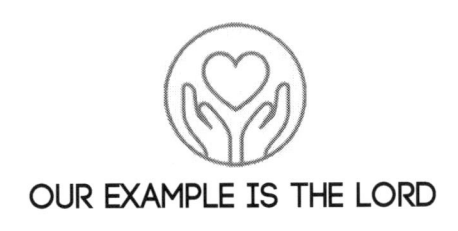

"'I will not look upon you in anger. For I am gracious,' declares the Lord; 'I will not be angry forever.'" Jeremiah 3:12b (NASV)

In this scripture, we get to see whom our God is, peaking behind the curtain. You know God is gracious and cares for you, but did you realize that God can and has gotten angry? We mostly see His anger displayed in the Old Testament. As a result of the Israelite's disobedience and turning to idol worship, He allowed them to be captured by the Assyrians and the Babylonians. In their captivity, their beloved Temple was destroyed. Recall that the Temple was the center of their worship and their existence; it was where God dwelled. Its destruction was a visible sign that God had departed them. Yet, we know He had not gone but was disciplining them for their disobedience. However, God had a way for them to be reconciled with Him. You nor I am God; therefore, who are we to be angry with individuals and try to extract punishment or vengeance? God is God, and He declares that He will not remain angry, so how can you?

Look upon God's example of being gracious and kind and extending mercy to those who hurt or wrong you. The way in which you care for your loved one will demonstrate whether you are allowing the character of God to shine through and shows that you have surrendered to His will.

REFLECTIONS:

- Am I a gracious person?
- Do I extend kindness to individuals?
- Do I accept people's apologies and extend a hand of forgiveness?
- Talk to your heavenly Father.

WHAT ARE YOU SAYING

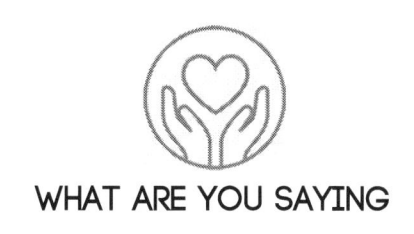

"A man's discretion makes him slow to anger, and it is his glory to overlook a transgression." Proverbs 19:11 (NASV)

We live in a society where we are encouraged to share everything. Social media has made it so easy to put our thoughts and emotions out for the entire world to see. Is this a good thing? Sometimes I think so but sometimes not. In this new season of your life, where it may be easier to share your frustrations, anger, and every detail of why this caregiving role isn't for you, it probably isn't productive...at least not yet. Today's scripture speaks to being discreet. Um, now that's a word we don't often hear! Being discreet is another way of saying being sensitive; with your words and actions, not displaying or revealing everything you are thinking or occurring in your life.

Think about how you speak to the person you care for. Perhaps your actions while caring for them may convey that you really don't want to be there and resent them. Maybe you give all the details of what it takes to care for them. Now please look at this from your loved one's point of view. Do you honestly think THEY wanted this for themselves? Do you think they want their business revealed to everyone? I think not, and your behavior around them is a constant reminder of THEIR current circumstance. No one wants to be totally dependent on another person. I urge you to look at what you say and how you say it, how to treat, bathe, and feed them. You change the environment by learning to be discreet with your words and behavior. Know that you have power in this season, and your behavior, thoughts, and comments will foster the environment in which you speak. Choose to overlook previous arguments, harsh words, or being absent from the relationship. Whatever the issue, CHOOSE to be discreet, and I will add, learn to forgive.

REFLECTIONS:

- What am I conveying as a caregiver?
- Is it loving or showing my anger?
- Talk with your heavenly Father.

WHO ARE YOUR FRIENDS

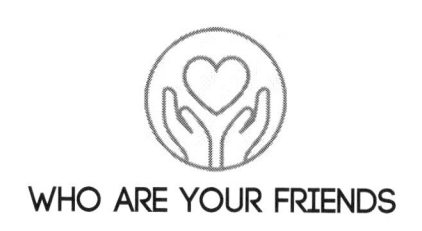

"Do not associate with a man given to anger, or go with a hot-tempered man." Proverbs 22:24 (NASV)

You have now taken on a role that will require ALL of you. It will not be easy, but it CAN be rewarding and joyful IF you let it. To help you in this role as a joyful caregiver, you must surround yourself with supportive family and friends. Although they may not be angry, they can be negative and consistently remind you what you are giving up and how hard this is on you. You don't need that; you need people who will comfort you and allow you the emotional freedom to be. Even though you may not be angry, you may find times when you are, and that's ok. That is the time for those supportive friends to lend a listening ear and allow you to cry, vent or eat a dozen cookies, but they will not bring it up once it's over. They will not recount all the reasons why this is so hard. They will listen, pray and eat cookies with you.

REFLECTIONS:

- Do I have a loving, supportive, and positive group of friends?
- How can I ensure I create an environment where I can draw supportive and positive friendships?
- Talk to the Father.

RELATIONSHIP IS EVERYTHING TO GOD

"But I say to you that everyone who is angry with his brother shall be guilty before the court; and whoever says to his brother, 'You good-for-nothing,' shall be guilty before the supreme court; and whoever says, 'You fool,' shall be guilty enough to go into the fiery hell. Therefore, if you are presenting your offering at the alter, and there remember that your brother has something against you, leave your offering there before the altar and go; first be reconciled to your brother, and then come and present your offering." Matthew 5:22-24 (NASV)

Scripture clearly shows that God expects us to live in harmony with one another. Living in harmony doesn't mean that you must always agree with an individual, comply with all their demands, or are always right. What it does mean is that there is a way to disagree and still be agreeable. God expects His children to be the first to extend the olive branch. Regardless of whether you feel it's your fault or the other person's, you are to do the forgiving and make the relationship right.

As you walk this caregiving journey, know that your anger can get in the way of God using you to display His love to the person you are caring for and as a public display to the world. Do not think for a second that people aren't watching you, especially if they know you are a believer. The world looks to us to see evidence of God, and when we slip up. I know that may sound strange, but it's true. How you care for your loved one brings glory to God and demonstrates your faith in Him to the world.

So, if you know there is someone to whom you need to apologize to, then do it! It's what God expects.

REFLECTIONS:

- Are there any strained relationships that I have?
- What must I do to make them right?
- Will I commit to bringing harmony to these relationships?
- Talk to your heavenly Father.

GOD'S GOT YOU

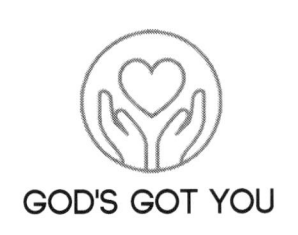

"Never take your own revenge, beloved, but leave room for the wrath of God, for it is written: 'Vengeance is Mine, I will repay,' says the Lord. 'But if your enemy is hungry, feed him; and if he is thirsty, give him a drink; for in so doing you will heap burning coals on his head. Do not be overcome by evil, but overcome evil with good.'" Romans 12:19-21 (NASV)

You may be tempted to take things into your own control, but is it wise? Today's scripture reminds us that God will ultimately repay us no matter our circumstances and how badly we have been treated. It isn't up to us to "punish" someone for their behavior. As you continue to care for your loved one, do not repay their harsh behavior with more harsh behavior. You are a child of the Most High God, and therefore you are to continue to do good and give God room to work in this situation. Trust me, you will come out the greater for it.

REFLECTIONS:

- Am I ready to let go and allow God to work in my heart?
- Do I trust God to let Him take control of this situation?
- Talk to your heavenly Father.

WHAT SHOULD YOU EXPECT

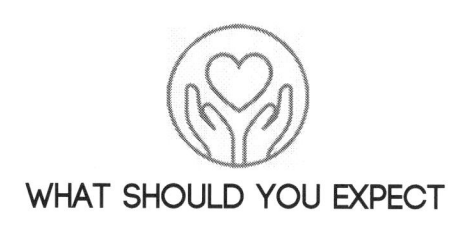

"But love your enemies, and do good, and lend, expecting nothing in return; and your reward will be great, and you will be sons of the Most High; for He Himself is kind to ungrateful and evil men." Luke 6:35 (NASV)

As a caregiver, your goal is to bring honor and glory to God. Let's face it, this is our daily goal whether we are caregivers or not. As children of God, everything we do can be, dare I say it should be, a way of honoring Him to bring honor and glory to His name. But in this season of caring, for some, this task becomes more heightened. Your daily challenges can often send you through the roof or exhaust you beyond comprehension! However, scripture shows that we are to expect NOTHING from being kind, extending a helping hand, and caring for an individual. Is this hard for you to hear? It was for me, at first, then as I grew with God during my caregiving season, I understood that I was to look toward God as my rewarder, and so should you. This season demonstrates how much you trust Him and how much you will look to Him to supply your needs. Are you expecting something from this season or from someone because you are a Christian? You know, walking in the fruit of the Spirit! Stop, and learn to expect nothing for your good deeds, at least from people. In this season, God is looking to see how much you trust Him. Will He find your faithfulness?

REFLECTIONS:

- Is God pleased with how I have cared for my loved one?
- Is my caregiving a reflection of the love God extends to me?
- Talk with your heavenly Father.

GOD'S GOT THIS

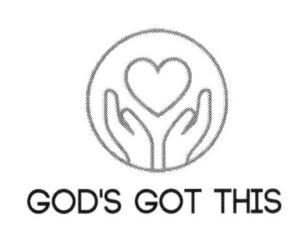

"God is a righteous judge, and a God who has indignation every day." Psalm 7:11 (NASV)

This may seem like a strange scripture, but it conveys how God restrains His own anger. Therefore, you can look to Him as a guide in handling situations that upset you—learning to release your anger because the wrong in your life will be made right in God's time. If you have or are harboring anger toward your loved one, give it to God. Know that whether your loved one shows it or not, they are hurting. No one would willingly plan to need a caregiver, to lose their autonomy and independence. Throughout this season, remember that God is a just and loving God. Although it may be difficult for you to see or feel His love during this time, IT IS THERE, and know that the hurt you've experienced by unkind acts, hurtful words that were spoken to you, and deliberate betrayals ALL have not gone unnoticed by God. In HIS time, He will bring justice. His indignation will not be restrained forever.

REFLECTIONS:

- What is it you want to release to the Lord?
- What hurtful situation or words do you wish God would bring justice to?
- Talk to your heavenly Father.

YOU'RE A BONDSERVANT FOR THE LORD

"But refuse foolish and ignorant speculations, knowing that they produce quarrels. The Lord's bond-servant must not be quarrelsome, but be kind to all, able to teach, patient when wronged," 2 Timothy 2:23-24 (NASB)

Did you realize you were God's bondservant? Whelp, you are. That is if you are a child of Christ. And I know you are. We are all bondservants, tied to our Master, Jesus. We belong to Him and are to reflect Him in all we do. As a young disciple, Paul's instruction to Timothy is to teach patience by being an example of patience, not to get into foolish arguments and discussions that lead to nowhere.

Think of the number of times you have engaged in what would be considered "foolish" discussions; discussions of you trying to win the argument or proving your point. Is this necessary from God's viewpoint? Probably not. It isn't important that you always be recognized as right but that within yourself, you know you are right. Having to prove your rightness leads to quarrels, and we see here that isn't what you, as a bondservant of the Lord, are to do.

REFLECTIONS:

- Must I always have the last word?
- Is it important to me to be recognized as being right?
- Must I prove my point to people?
- Talk with your heavenly Father.

REFLECTIONS
ACTION STEPS
PRAYERS

CHAPTER THREE
Fear and Worry

Although scripture tells us not to be anxious about anything, the reality is that we, as children of God, still become fearful and anxious. The world can be a scary place especially when you're suddenly put in the role of caregiver for a spouse, parent, and/or sibling. The fears of how you will manage could take over; fears of financial burdens, juggling other family responsibilities, our emotions, etc. But they do not have to. The following devotions will help you manage the fear.

WHAT ARE YOU AFRAID OF

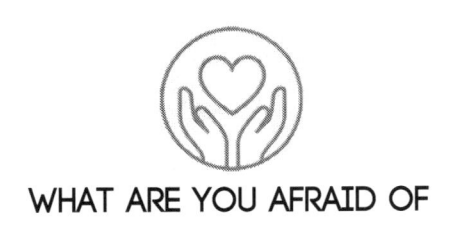

> "The Lord is my light and my salvation—whom should I fear?
> The Lord is the stronghold of my life—whom should I dread?"
> Psalm 27:1 (CSB)

Being a caregiver can be pretty scary. You get to witness the advancement of your loved one's disease as it erases the person you knew them to be. You get to experience what it is like to see someone suffer and be helpless without real relief. Yes, as the caregiver, YOU get to minister and cater to them daily, sometimes not receiving a break or a thank you. You get to witness the inevitable loss of your loved one. All caregiving is scary, but you do not have to walk in fear or denial. David, in this Psalm, was being attacked and pursued by Saul. You are being pursued by an enemy who wants to destroy you and take your strength. However, he can only succeed if you forget who you are and where you draw your power from. God is your stronghold, your light, and God is in this season right with you. Don't allow the enemy to bombard you with worry that renders your mind and actions stagnate. You are a child of the Most High God, and He will not fail you.

REFLECTIONS:
- What am I afraid of? Be honest.
- Do I believe God can overcome what I am afraid of?

PRAYER:

Lord, I'm scared. I never saw this coming and don't want to go through this. However, I put my trust in You. So, if this season is what You have for me, I embrace it with You—knowing that You will help me. I ask that You help me not walk in fear, worry, or dread. Please help me to see Your good works because I know You are working on my behalf and my loved one. Please help me to trust You daily and to surrender to You daily. And help my life bring honor and glory to Your name. In Jesus' Name, Amen!

CRIPPLED BY FEAR

"For God has not given us a spirit of fear, but one of power, love, and sound judgment." 2 Timothy 1:7 (CSV)

Has your recent thrust into caregiving led you down a road of doom and fear? It can be terrifying to look at all that is required of you and the fate of your loved one, BUT is fear from God? No! The enemy uses fear to keep us (you) from trusting in the Lord, to keep you off track. Once you continue to look at the "problem" and see that there appears to be one road ahead, YOU STAY right where you are, not making any progress. Your God is a forward-looking God who sees where you are and where HE wants you to go. However, to go where He has destined, you must trust Him and get your sights on Him. Believe that He has given YOU the power to do precisely what is needed this season and move FORWARD with love and sound judgment.

ACTION STEPS:

- Consciously think of what has been on your mind. Is it a lot of what "needs" to be done, or is it more of "I can't imagine how I will get through this?" Perhaps it's both. Jot down what has been on your mind. Then list how God is providing for you. Which list is longer?
- If the "needs" list or "I can't imagine how..." list is longer than how God is providing for you, you may be crippled by fear and worry. In either case, this is not of God.
- Take a moment to remember that you are not alone and that God has given YOU the power to endure and overcome this.

PRAYER:

Dear Lord, I acknowledge that I am fearful, fearful about if all of this will work out, fearful of whether I can emotionally, physically, and financially handle this, and fearful of the loss of my loved one and myself. I know fear doesn't come from You but from the enemy. Today I declare that I will walk in power and love, and make sound decisions. I'll take one day at a time with You. I am seeking Your guidance and constant fellowship. I know that You have already solved all of the issues I will face today and tomorrow, but I will now focus on today and allow You to direct me. I put my complete trust in You. Thank You for loving me and providing for me. In Jesus' Name, I pray, Amen.

AN ANXIOUS MIND

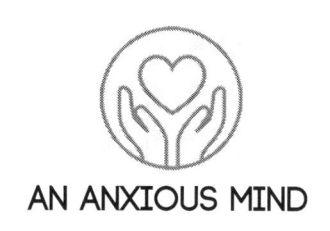

"How long, Lord? Will you forget me forever? How long will you hide your face from me? How long will I store up anxious concerns within me, agony in my mind every day? How long will my enemy dominate me? Consider me and answer, Lord my God. Restore brightness to my eyes; otherwise, I will sleep in death. My enemy will say, 'I have triumphed over him,' and my foes will rejoice because I am shaken. But I have trusted in your faithful love; my heart will rejoice in your deliverance. I will sing to the Lord because he has treated me generously." Psalm 13 (CSB)

We can use many examples from David's life to emulate and those we should not. Today we concentrate on how very transparent David was with God. He exposes his heart and what's on his mind. In this Psalm, we see David is troubled; he has anxious thoughts and for a good reason. King Saul wanted him dead and was pursuing him to kill him! I guess everyone would have anxious thoughts about that!

What are your anxious thoughts now that you are a caregiver? Are they ideas about what will happen tomorrow or the news you're expecting to get today? Dear heart, as you read this passage, look at how David voices his concern. Initially, he accuses God of forgetting him; then, he confesses that he is worried and perhaps a little scared. He recounts, as if God was clueless, that he is being hunted down like an animal and that those who hunt him will delight in his capture. After unloading his heart, he turns to what he truly knows. He remembers that God equipped him to defeat Goliath and that he killed both a bear and a lion when he was a shepherd. This walk down memory lane puts him back into a mindset of worship and praise. He declares he will continue to trust the Lord and changes his thoughts about what is currently happening to what he knows will happen, which causes him to worship and praise the Lord.

ACTION STEPS:

- Reread this psalm out loud. Then insert your own words. Example "How long will I continue to wrestle with MEDICARE, MEDICAID, or how long will my sibling(s) continue to fight me or will my loved one suffer?"
- Write your verse. Read it aloud, and add the last part, "But I have trusted in Your faithful love; my heart will rejoice in Your deliverance. I will sing to the Lord because he has treated me generously," and recite that again until you truly recognize that you can trust God and that He has been and will continue to be generous toward you.

FEAR OF THE FUTURE

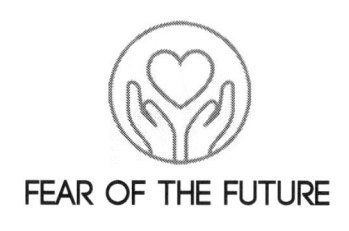

"'For I know the plans I have for you' - this is the Lord's declaration - 'plans for your well-being, not for disaster, to give you a future and a hope.'" Jeremiah 29:11 (CSV)

Looking ahead can often steal today's joys while simultaneously slowing us down to what must be done today to ensure tomorrow is good. God has declared that He has a good plan for you! It is your responsibility to BELIEVE HIM. Looking at your circumstances and listening to others' perceptions and "advice" can often distract you from what God says. Your future is secure in Him. This season is part of your future. God is using all of your circumstances, including this season of caregiving, to guide you toward His desired path...you must choose to trust Him and follow. Rest in His word.

REFLECTIONS:

- Do you want to be satisfied with what life may look like in the future?
- Do you think many of your dreams and/or aspirations still need to be attainable?

ACTION STEPS:

- Jot down everything you were "going to do" before caregiving. Then reassess what can still be done, perhaps with some modifications, what may need to be postponed, and finally, what is no longer an option.
- Focus on those things that you can do and prioritize. Then create or add those things that must wait until later to your bucket list.
- Finally, thank God for showing you that all is not lost and for giving you new dreams, goals, and a promising future.

FEARING THE WORST

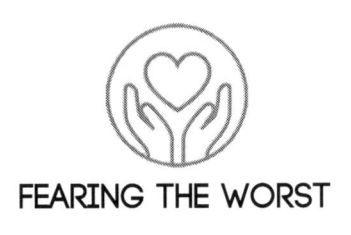

"Hallelujah! I will praise the Lord with all my heart in the assembly of the upright and in the congregation. The Lord's works are great, studied by all who delight in them. All that he does is splendid and majestic; his righteousness endures forever. He has caused his wondrous works to be remembered. The Lord is gracious and compassionate. He has provided food for those who fear him; he remembers his covenant forever. He has shown his people the power of his works by giving them the inheritance of the nations. The works of his hands are truth and justice; all his instructions are trustworthy. They are established forever and ever, enacted in truth and in uprightness. He has sent redemption to his people. He has ordained his covenant forever. His name is holy and awe-inspiring. The fear of the Lord is the beginning of wisdom; all who follow his instructions have good insight. His praise endures forever." Psalm 111 (CSB)

There are those days when you know something terrible will happen, or it has already happened, and you've internalized it, living with it daily. And you ask, "How much can one person be expected to take?" Remember that although you are going through a tough life, it will not crush you. God knows EXACTLY what you can handle. Caregiving can be a tough time, and the fact that you have been called to caregiving means you will get through it! However, you choose how you will get through it. Today you will focus on looking at ALL God has done for you. Stop concentrating on the bad and focus on what you know about God. God is good and faithful and will never leave you or forsake you.

ACTION STEPS:

- Read today's scriptures out loud with intensity and full of joy.
- That is how you counter fear with worship and praise to the Lord!

DON'T GET AHEAD OF YOURSELF

"Therefore, don't worry about tomorrow, because tomorrow will worry about itself. Each day has enough trouble of its own."
Matthew 6:34 (CSV)

Each day is filled with both good and bad, with thousands of choices and decisions to be made every day. Often, we begin to think past today and look toward the next day, then the next. Then you find your mind has taken you to a year out. What will happen, how can I cope, how will I manage? Jesus provides the remedy for this mind-wandering. It's simple, just concentrate on TODAY! I can hear you saying, "It's easier said than done!" You are right, but it can be done. It will take concentration on your part, and you will fail a couple of times before you "master" it, but it can be done.

Why do you think this is in scripture? Could it be that by focusing on the "future," we neglect what must be done today? I believe that is part of it. Also, the truth is that you don't know what tomorrow will look like, so how can you effectively plan for it...without God. Jesus instructs you to concentrate on today because today is what you can handle. He's got tomorrow, and when tomorrow comes, you will be able to tackle those issues then.

REFLECTIONS:

- How do you get ahead of yourself?
- Are you a procrastinator because today's tasks seem too daunting?

ACTION STEPS:

- Make a list of those things that MUST be done today.
- Make another list of those things that CAN be done today.
- Make another list of those things that you would LIKE to do today.
- Pray over all lists, then start your day by doing the list that MUST be done. Once completed, tackle the list that CAN be done, followed by what you'd LIKE to do.
- Don't sweat it if you don't complete the first list. Life happens, but at least you DID achieve something. The next day, reassess the remaining items on the list, add what needs to be done that day, and start anew. Someday you may make it to your "like" to-do list. On other days, you may even complete those items on the "like-to-accomplish" list. Some days, you will not even tackle the items on the MUST be done list. It's ok. There's always tomorrow.

WORRYING...WASTING TIME

> "Can any of you add one moment to his life span by worrying?"
> Matthew 6:27 (CSB)

Well, can you? Can your worry about this season of caretaking actually add an extra day or ensure a better outcome? The answer is NO. You have not been called to worry about life but to live the life God has given you. Worrying robs you of seeing all the amazing things God is doing RIGHT NOW in this season. Worrying keeps your focus on the circumstances, which is the opposite of what God calls us to do. Instead, He tells us to look at things through the lens of eternity. Translation, get your mind off you and put it on Him. He is the One who is the actual "change agent." This season will become more manageable by placing your trust and consistently focusing on Him. Listen, I truly believe what God tells us in His word. If you're going through something difficult, then it means He has given you the grace and strength to endure and complete it with victory. You may have to align your definition of "victory" with His but trust me; you can do this!

ACTION STEPS:

- List everything that you are worried about. Everything!
- With your list in hand, tell the Lord. Go over what is on the list, and after you have prayed about it, tear the list up and throw it away! You have just given everything to God, and now He is responsible. You are to trust Him. As the anxiety creeps back into your mind, because it will, visualize you throwing that lists away and remind yourself, "God's got it," then say aloud, "Thank you, Lord, for taking care of this situation."

WHAT TO DO WHEN YOU'RE AFRAID

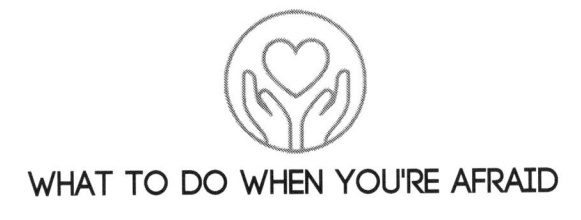

> "When I am afraid, I will trust in you. In God, whose word I praise, in God I trust; I will not be afraid. What can mere mortals do to me?" Psalm 56:3-4 (CSV)

This new season will be scary; at least it was for me. I had never cared for anyone, and the weight of the responsibility of caring for my mother, who was diagnosed with Alzheimer's, sent shock waves through me. But as the Psalmist wrote, I did. I put my trust in God and encourage you to do the same.

Through this season of caregiving, as you trust God more, you will develop a lovely, intimate relationship with Him. He will guide you and comfort you. The Holy Spirit will guide you and show you what to do and how. God will put people in your path to assist you and provide sound counsel. And most of all, He will surround you with His love. Yes, caregiving will be scary but put your trust in God and then marvel at how He makes way for you!

ACTION STEPS:

- Throughout the day, say aloud, "I put my trust in God; therefore, I am not afraid."

PRAYER:

Dear Lord, I am afraid of my loved one dying; fearful of all that I may lose in my life as I take responsibility for my loved one's care; worried that I may make a mistake or a wrong decision; afraid of financial ruin, and just scared. But I will put my trust in You because I know that You are the One who loves me and cares for me. I don't understand why this season fell upon me and my loved one, but I choose this day to TRUST YOU and HONOR YOU with my service. I am not afraid! In Jesus' Name, Amen.

BE NOT AFRAID

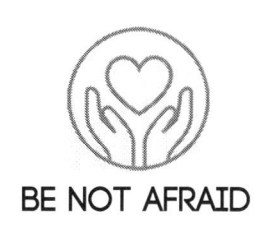

"Haven't I commanded you: be strong and courageous? Do not be afraid or discouraged, for the Lord your God is with you wherever you go." Joshua 1:9 (CSV)

Listen to what God is telling YOU. Just as He commanded Joshua after he assumed leadership of the newly founded nation of Israel, He also commands YOU to be strong and courageous. He reminds you that He is with you and will be with you throughout this season. Knowing that your Creator is with you should provide the peace and assurance you need to take each day, one day at a time.

See, God knows that this walk will not be easy, but with Him, you can be assured that you will walk through this season with victory and joy.

REFLECTIONS:

- How does this season scare you?
- Do you consider yourself to be courageous? Why or why not?
- Know that God does see you as courageous.
- Talk to your heavenly Father.

FEAR GOD AND HAVE PEACE

> "You who fear the Lord, trust in the Lord! He is their help and shield." Psalm 115:11 (CSV)

The one thing I really want you to understand, believe, and know is that you can trust God!!! He is there right with you as you embark on this caregiving journey. The journey may be a long one that will test you and exhaust all of your emotions, or it may be a short one where you're left short-changed. Either one is horrible and hard to endure but know that YOU can Trust God!!! He is the same God you find in the Old Testament who led the Israelites out of Egypt; the same God who is so holy. It is remarkable that He loves us at all! Yet He does, and He loves YOU!!

Go to Him and talk with Him and worship His Holy Name. Learn to delight yourself in Him, and I assure you peace will follow.

ACTION STEPS:

- Find your favorite song or hymn. One perhaps you recall from your childhood or the hymn sung the first time you accepted Christ. Then go to a nice quiet place where you are all alone and sing it! Yes, sing it out loud...Jesus thinks you have an incredible voice. Sing and then tell the Lord how much you love Him. After that, tell Him what's on your heart and that you need Him.

NO FEAR

"Surely the righteous will never be shaken; they will be remembered forever. They will have no fear of bad news; their hearts are steadfast, trusting in the Lord." Psalm 112:6-7 (NIV)

As a child of God, fear isn't something you have inherited from your heavenly Father; fear comes from the enemy. Not having a solid relationship with God and knowing who you are in Him will allow you to experience fear. I'm not defining fear as merely being afraid of something but the fear that keeps you in one place; it hinders you from moving forward. That fear is precisely what the enemy wants... you not to move forward. Yet God has ordered your steps and has created a path for you to follow. See the choice you must make? Trust God and move forward!

REFLECTIONS:

- Are you afraid of moving forward, of the future? Why?
- Talk with your heavenly Father.

STOP WORRYING AND START PRAYING

> "Don't worry about anything, but in everything, through prayer and petition with thanksgiving; present your requests to God. And the peace of God, which surpasses all understanding, will guard your hearts and minds in Christ Jesus."
> Philippians 4:6-7 (CSB)

Not being anxious is pretty simple, right...perhaps not. This season has so many twists and turns, and ups and downs. You have your good days, then maybe a great day gets in there somewhere, but many days are routine, perhaps dull, and then there are those that are so scary that they shock you to your core. What are you to do with all your anxiety, concerns about what to do next, and "what if's?" Well, sweet one, you bundle up all of it. Your nerves are just about to erupt into who knows what, you're foreboding of the future, and go to God. I mean, immediately go to Him. Once you start to feel nervous about a situation, go to Him. Once you think that you are at the end of your last nerve, go to Him. And this is what you say when you go to God, "HELP." It is that simple. You ask the One who truly loves you for help. And guess what? He will. That is the peace that Paul refers to in our scripture for today. Once you go to God and admit you can't handle it, that you need His guidance and intervention, you will experience peace. You won't be able to explain it...not rationally, because your problems won't instantaneously disappear. They'll linger for a while. But you will know that you are not doing this alone. You have God almighty on your side, bringing peace.

ACTION STEPS:

- Go into a quiet room, sit, and think of all you must do today. Do you feel yourself getting a little anxious? Then STOP and say, "Help me, Lord, I need You today." Then have a little talk with Jesus.

- When you get a chance, I would encourage you to read the verses to the hymn, "Have a Little Talk with Jesus." Concentrate on the chorus and allow it to strengthen your soul and take away all of your fears and worries.

WHERE IS YOUR FAITH

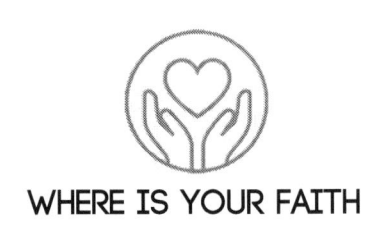

"One day he and his disciples got into a boat, and he told them, 'Let's cross over to the other side of the lake.' So they set out, and as they were sailing he fell asleep. Then a fierce windstorm came down on the lake; they were being swamped and were in danger. They came and woke him up, saying, 'Master, Master, we're going to die!' Then he got up and rebuked the wind and the raging waves. So they ceased, and there was a calm. He said to them, 'Where is your faith?' They were fearful and amazed, asking one another, 'Who then is this? He commands even the winds and the waves, and they obey him!'" Luke 8:22-25 (CSB)

The disciples were scared! They were so scared that they forgot who they were in the boat with and so frightened that they forgot that it was Jesus' idea! Had Jesus made a statement in the past that had not occurred? No, Jesus always said what He meant and meant what He said. Yet here they are, scared! At least they didn't worry; instead, they woke Jesus up. And after confessing their fear and accusing Him of not caring, Jesus gets up and stops the storm. Then He asked the question, "Where is your faith?" Another translation, "Why can't you trust me?" WOW, I wonder how they felt when He asked that question. The scripture does not indicate that it had any impact because the disciples focused on Jesus stopping the storm and His authority to such. I think it went right over their heads. But do not let Jesus' question go over your head. Where is your faith? This time is tough, and there will be days when you want to give in…but remember Jesus is in the boat with you! Believe it or not, when you accepted Him as your Savior, He climbed into your lifeboat and called you to go to the other side with Him. Yes, there will be storms but know you will get to the other side.

REFLECTIONS:

- Where is my faith?

PRAYER:

Lord, I admit that I am very scared. Being a caregiver is hard, and watching my loved one suffer is even more challenging. I don't understand why this is the particular path You have chosen for me and my loved one, but I will trust You. I know that You are here with me and that if I continue to put my trust in You and commit daily to fellowship with You, I will make it. This day Lord, I choose to walk by faith!

LEAN ON GOD

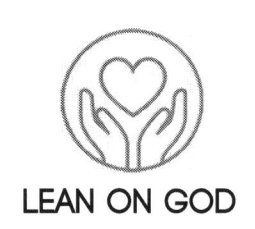

> "Do not fear, for I am with you; do not be afraid, for I am your God. I will strengthen you; I will help you; I will hold on to you with my righteous right hand." Isaiah 41:10 (CSV)

How awesome to know that God is holding you up right this very second. Do you know this? The God of the universe is right there with you, holding onto you as if for dear life. Why? Because He knows you can't do it yourself and because He loves you and wants to be close to you. Do not allow the enemy to tell you any different. There is no need to fear because YOUR God is with you.

ACTION STEPS:

- Meditate on this scripture throughout the day. When you feel anxious or nervous, remember this scripture, and say it aloud. And remember, you are never alone!

THE SOURCE OF YOUR STRENGTH

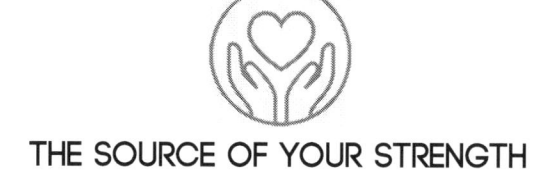

> "I lift my eyes toward the mountains. Where will my help come from? My help comes from the Lord, the Maker of heaven and earth." Psalm 121:1-2 (CSB)

You may not know this, but you do have the strength to make it through this season. You have the power to continue this caregiving journey with joy and peace. As you continue this journey, you must rely on God. It is through His strength that you find your own. Today's scripture points your focus back to God and off of your circumstances. Too often, your focus is on the problems and daily grind that must be accomplished. But God wants you to focus on Him. When you look at the world around you, the beauty of creation testifies to God's greatness and goodness.

The Creator of all that created YOU has not left you alone. He is your strength and helps every day of your life. He created you for fellowship with Him, to delight in Him, and to go through life with Him. Today, rest and look up and see the majesty and strength of your God!

REFLECTIONS:

- What frustrates you?
- Within 24 hours, how much time do you spend fretting or worrying about your circumstance?

ACTION STEPS:

- The amount of time you spend worrying is the exact amount of time you will now spend in prayer and studying God's word. As a recommendation for study, begin with the Proverbs. Read one chapter a day and then pray to the Lord. Your worrying will decrease as you grow in His word and fellowship with Him more.

YOU ARE STRONG

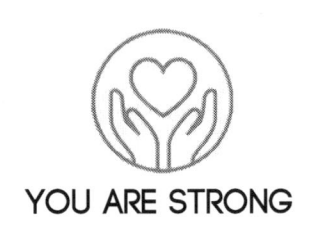

> "Be strong and courageous; don't be terrified or afraid of them. For the Lord your God is the one who will go with you; he will not leave you or abandon you." Deuteronomy 31:6 (CSV)

You may not realize it, but you are strong. Want to know how I know? Because you have the Almighty on your side!!! You have the advantage in every event that occurs in your life. Yes, I know it may not look like you have the edge, but you do. Nowhere in the Bible will you find it written that life is all roses and unicorns for Christians. Nowhere, yet we are to rejoice! Why? Because we have Christ who came and reconciled us back to God, we can have an open and honest dialog with Him any time through that reconciliation. It is your relationship with God that gives you the advantage! He is always going to do what is right and just, always. Your role is to trust Him.

ACTION STEPS:

- Go to the mirror, look at yourself, and then recite Deuteronomy 31:6, as I have written below, for you to insert yourself into the scripture. Do it as many times as you need to start believing it!

PRAYER:

I am strong and courageous, not terrified or afraid of anyone. For the Lord MY God is the One who will go with me; He will not leave me or abandon me!

YOU ARE NOT ALONE

"The Lord is for me; I will not be afraid. What can a mere mortal do to me? The Lord is my helper; therefore, I will look in triumph on those who hate me." Psalm 118:6-7 (CSV)

Do you realize that God is for YOU? The God of the universe, creator of heaven and earth, who formed you in your mother's womb, IS FOR YOU? He is on YOUR side and wants you to have a good outcome. He wants you to know that nothing can harm you once you put your complete trust in Him. He is YOUR helper!

Now the enemy will try you, placing obstacles in your way, but once you have planted your flag in the Jesus camp, the enemy is rendered helpless. Oh, he still tries, BUT with the confidence and assurance you have in fully embracing that God is on your side, you can go boldly and do whatever is needed to take care of the person God has given you charge over.

PRAYER:

Dear Lord, it is hard for me to believe that You are on my side, but You are, so thank You. Lord being a caregiver is hard, and I need help. I ask that You work within me to allow Your Spirit to fill me and instruct me in what I need to do to ensure my loved one has the best care possible and that my season of caregiving brings honor and glory to Your Name. Please teach me how to walk with the assurance of Your presence and provision in this season. In Jesus' Name, Amen.

YOU CAN DO THIS

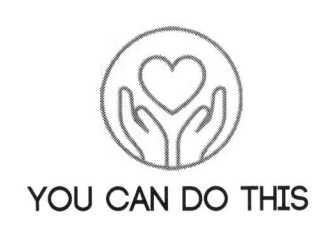

"Then David said to his son Solomon, 'Be strong and courageous, and do the work. Don't be afraid or discouraged, for the Lord God, my God, is with you. He won't leave you or abandon you until all the work for the service of the Lord's house is finished.'"
1 Chronicles 28:20 (CSV)

Dear one, this season will require a lot from you, but know that the 'Lord God, My God, is with YOU.' These are the words David is giving his son, which I also give to YOU because you need to know that YOU CAN DO THIS! The reason is that God is with YOU!! As you learn to trust Him and go to Him with everything in your heart and the things you have accomplished daily, you'll discover you can handle this season.

This first part of David's advice stresses, 'do the work,' meaning there will be work for you to do as a caregiver and so many things to check off your daily "To Do" list, for example, feeding your loved one, perhaps toileting your loved one, contacting the doctor, medication management, supervising an outside caregiver, running the home, the children, your job, etc. So many things to do, but you are to DO THE WORK. Why? Let's look at the latter portion of David's advice to his son. Take a close look at the last sentence of David's advice. God will be with you as you DO THE WORK for the service of the Lord's house. Now you aren't building a temple, but your life and the life of your loved one bring honor and glory to God. Your season of caregiving is a service to the Lord. I want you to think about that for a minute. How you care for your loved one either brings honor to God or dishonors God. Never forget that as a believer, everything you do is a witness to your relationship with God. Yes, everything, including caregiving. But God never gives you more than you can bear, so rest in knowing that He is with you, and you can do the work!

ACTION STEPS (1):

- Take time to meditate on your caregiving as a service to the Lord.

REFLECTIONS:

- Now that you know your caregiving is a service to the Lord, is there anything you must change to ensure your service honors the Lord?

ACTION STEPS (2):

- Implement the changes you have identified above.

YOU BELONG TO THE LORD

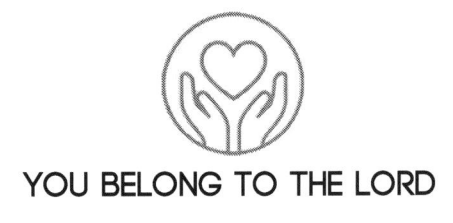

"Now this is what the Lord says - the one who created you, Jacob, and the one who formed you, Israel – 'Do not fear, for I have redeemed you; I have called you by your name; you are mine. When you pass through the waters, I will be with you, and the rivers will not overwhelm you. When you walk through the fire, you will not be scorched, and the flame will not burn you. For I am the Lord your God, the Holy One of Israel, and your Savior. I have given Egypt as a ransom for you, Cush and Seba in your place. Because you are precious in my sight and honored, and I love you, I will give people in exchange for you and nations instead of your life.'" Isaiah 43:1-4 (CSB)

What a powerful statement God makes to those who choose to follow Him. You, dear heart, have chosen to follow Him; therefore, you are His. Today I want you to reflect on His love letter to YOU. Don't be confused with the references to Jacob and Israel; you are a part of that called-out nation. The enemies of their day were the other nations. Your enemies are different, but the words from the Lord are the same to you. He loves you. Because of His love, you do not need to worry or be disheartened.

ACTION STEPS:

- I want you to look in the mirror and repeat: "Because I am precious to the Lord; because He loves ME, I will trust Him."
- Do this out loud in the morning, at lunch, and before you go to bed.

WILL THINGS GET BETTER

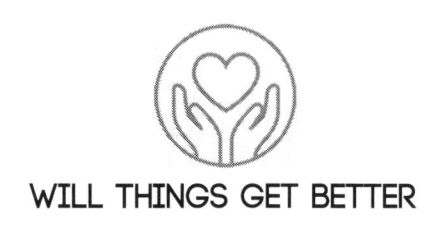

"We know that all things work together for the good of those who love God, who are called according to his purpose."
Romans 8:28 (CSB)

Do you love the Lord? Another way to ask this question is, are you actively following His word? Are you trying to learn more and more about Him? Have you dedicated your life to Him? If yes, then you love the Lord. Our scripture today shows us that those who love God and are called according to His purpose will see how He maneuvers your life events to work out for YOUR good. It isn't essential right now that you see things working out for your good, but that you KNOW that things will work out for your good. Do you believe it? Do you trust God and take Him at His word? The answer has to be YES!!! You will never get all the answers to why you are experiencing life in the way you are. Still, you can rest in knowing that as long as you Love God (following His word, fellowship with Him daily, making Him a priority in your life, and seeking His counsel), things will work out for YOUR good and for His glory.

ACTION STEPS:

- Commit to making God THE priority in your life. That doesn't mean that you neglect your responsibilities. It means you set aside time in your day to read God's word (as you are doing now) and then talk with Him and seek His counsel. Do it daily and begin to hear Him speak to you. The Holy Spirit will guide you through this season. He will lead you to the answers you need.

ARE YOU FRUITFUL OR ARE YOU WORRYING

> "Others are like seed sown among thorns; these are the ones who hear the word, but the worries of this age, the deceitfulness of wealth, and the desires for other things enter in and choke the word, and it becomes unfruitful." Mark 4:18-19 (CSB)

This is taken from the parable Jesus taught of the sower of the seed, highlighting how people receive God's word. Most Christians think this strictly refers to unbelievers, which is true, but it must continue to speak to us, you, the Christians. You are still in the process of growing and hearing the word of God. How are you receiving it? Today's scripture shows that worry can block you from hearing and seeing God! I know it may be redundant, but so what? Keeping your focus on God allows you to grow in Him. The contrast is having a mind full of worry, constantly looking at the world, things that are going on in your life, and the daily challenges that you must face. Notice that the scripture isn't telling you to ignore your circumstances but to not focus on them. Worrying is consistent daily, every minute, concentrating on something difficult. It chokes your mind from seeing God and then realizing that He will help you, and with God's help, you become fruitful, living the life He has equipped you to live. So, you have a decision to make; you can trust God or worry, but you cannot do both!

REFLECTIONS:

- Am I a worrier, or do I trust in God's sovereign plan and protection in my life?
- Talk with your heavenly Father.

A COVENANT OF PEACE

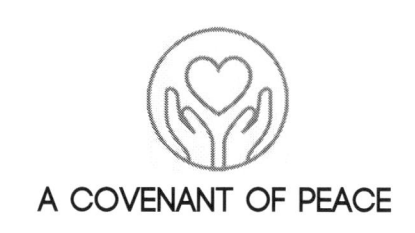

"For the mountains may depart, and the hills be removed; but my lovingkindness shall not depart from thee, neither shall my covenant of peace be removed, saith Jehovah that hath mercy on thee." Isaiah 54:10 (ASV)

Often you will be faced with overwhelming decisions, differences of opinion, and starts and stops, but in all of this, you are to have peace. Peace is the gauge in which you will know that you are walking in the will of God. If you embark on a decision in which you do not have peace, then that is the Holy Spirit's way of telling you not to do it. God gives us His peace, and this scripture shows that He has established a covenant of peace with YOU.

Worry and fretting aren't of God. Peace is of God. He loves you and is here for you during this season. His lovingkindness toward you means you aren't alone. He has made a way and loves you. Doesn't that bring peace to your soul? Rest in it.

ACTION STEPS:

- Today I want you to look in the mirror and say: "God loves me."
- Now, say it again like you believe it, "GOD LOVES ME!"
- Then one more time, as if announcing to the world, "GOD LOVES ME!!"
- If this doesn't bring peace, then repeat until it does.

RESTING IN GOD'S CARE

"The Lord is my shepherd; I have what I need. He lets me lie down in green pastures; he leads me beside quiet waters. He renews my life; he leads me along the right paths for his name's sake. Even when I go through the darkest valley, I fear no danger, for you are with me; your rod and your staff - they comfort me. You prepare a table before me in the presence of my enemies; you anoint my head with oil; my cup overflows. Only goodness and faithful love will pursue me all the days of my life, and I will dwell in the house of the Lord as long as I live." Psalm 23 (CSB)

Psalm 23 is a very familiar scripture! It is often recited from memory and has eased many believers' angst. Today, I want you to read this familiar scripture with new eyes. Read it out loud and allow each sentence to resonate within you. Each time you read a sentence, pause, and think about what it is saying to you and how you can apply it to your life right now and write it down! At the end of the scripture, look back and see how God has and will continue to be your provider, healer, strength, and comforter. Then rejoice!

REFLECTIONS
ACTION STEPS
PRAYERS

CHAPTER FOUR

Loneliness

Throughout my caregiving journey, I experienced times of loneliness. I felt isolated and alone as I cared for my mother, not because friends or family had abandoned me, which they did not, but because I was losing my mother. The loneliness of realizing that the one person who truly loved me unconditionally here on earth was disappearing. The woman I knew was leaving. She could no longer engage in conversations with me. We could no longer experience a movie, and I missed her laughter and smile. No one could change that or make that realization better.

I have no idea what may cause you to experience loneliness during your caregiving season. Know that God is always with you, and therefore you are not alone.

Allow these devotionals to help you know how much you are valued and loved.

HAVING A PITY PARTY ARE WE

"Look to the right and see: no one stands up for me; there is no refuge for me; no one cares about me." Psalm 142:4 (CSB)

I don't think anyone can throw a better pity than I can! Boy, I mean a full-blown party complete with tears, a runny nose, and the deep sense that "no one cares about me!" Yep, that's what I did through the first part of my caregiving journey. Are you throwing a pity party? I recall someone stating that pity parties weren't good parties because there is never any food, and no one ever comes! In truth, we don't want anyone to come. We prefer to wallow in our misery of being lonely. I caution you not to do this. A pity party takes the focus away from God and puts the focus on YOU. Our flesh would like to make us believe that everything that happens to you in this life is about YOU, but the word of God suggests differently. See…it's all about Him, Jesus, and what He did for you AND what He wants to do for others within your circle of influence through YOU! God wants to use YOU to draw others closer to Him. This season is just a part of that journey for you. So cut down on the pity parties. Dry your eyes, blow your nose, and know that the ONE Person you truly need to care about you DOES. His Name is Jesus!

REFLECTIONS:
- How many pity parties have you had?
- Describe what one of them looks like.
- Talk with your heavenly Father (share your loneliness with Him).

DOES ANYONE CARE

"Turn to me and be gracious to me, for I am alone and afflicted. The distresses of my heart increase; bring me out of my sufferings." Psalm 25:16-17 (CSV)

Our brother David is in distress and in need of God's comfort. He asked that God deliver him from his suffering. As a caregiver, the journey of caregiving can be considered suffering. It was for me as I watched the woman who gave birth to me slowly disappear. Toward the end of her season with Alzheimer's, I could tell she no longer recognized me as her daughter. I hurt for the mother I had and hurt for the woman before me. I aimed to ensure that she did not feel threatened by me but that I became a familiar and reassuring face. This was the one aspect of my caregiving journey where I felt alone and sometimes lost. My distress was palpable.

For many other reasons, caregiving can be a lonely period. However, it doesn't have to be lonely and isolating the entire journey. Like me, as you gain more and more confidence in your ability as a caregiver and continue to surrender to God and run to Him with your distress and feelings of loneliness, God gently guides you through. The loneliness decreases, and you find yourself being able to place one foot in front of the other. God brings people in and out of your life to help you and provide comfort and laughter.

It never will get "easy," but it will be easier. Your journey in this season is to put your complete trust in God. Allow Him to guide you and lavish you with love. As you grow in Him, you will also grow in your ability to caretake, and over time you will look back and see how far you have come and that you were never alone!

PRAYER:

Dear Lord, I pray for my dear friend as they embark on this caregiving journey. Help them to know that they are not alone and that You care so much for them. I ask that they feel Your peace. Grant them rest and surround them with individuals who will intercede for them and embrace and encourage them along this journey. Help them to know that You are with them. In Jesus' Name, Amen.

CRYING IS THERAPEUTIC

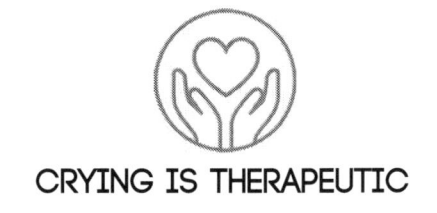

"Lord, God of my salvation, I cry out before you day and night. May my prayer reach your presence; listen to my cry."
Psalm 88:1-2 (CSB)

I know you've heard this before, but it is so true. Crying is one way the body decompresses from stress. So, have you had a good cry yet, or are you like David in today's scripture? You are just about all cried out! Well, dear heart, I hate to be the one to tell you, but as you continue in this season, you will have days where you don't feel the need to cry, then there will be days when you do! Embrace both! But as you cry, know that God is right there with you. Your tears touch His heart, and He knows and understands the pain and anguish you are going through. Remember, He voluntarily gave His Son to die on the cross for YOU. He watched as His Son was crucified, and He watched it because He knew that was the only way to allow YOU to have full access to Him. You were worth that!!! So, as you shed tears of frustration, anger, or despair, remember that God loves you, hears your pleas, and will never leave or forsake you. You are His and His alone!

REFLECTIONS:

- Take a moment to reflect on how much God loves you.
- List all the things in your life that reflect His love for you.
- Talk with your heavenly Father (tell Him how much you love Him).

EVEN THOUGH FAMILY MAY ABANDON YOU, YOU AREN'T ALONE

> "You've always been right there for me; don't turn your back on me now. Don't throw me out, don't abandon me; you've always kept the door open. My father and mother walked out and left me, but God took me in." Psalm 27:9-10 (The Message)

Caregiving will not only show you what you are made of, but it will also reveal or further expose the strength of your relationships, whether those relationships are with family or friends. As you learn to put the needs of your loved one first, you may encounter pushback. Sometimes the pushback may be well-meaning, but if the pushback comes from people who aren't willing to help you, you must learn to remain focused on what God has told YOU to do. In doing so, you may find that family and/or friends will so disagree with you that they stop being civil.

You may be left alone, but today's scripture shows that God is and will always be right by your side, even if those closest to you leave.

PRAYER:

Dear Lord, I know You are guiding me and with me. I ask that You give me the strength to make the right decisions for my loved one and me. I thank You for taking care of our needs. I lift up my family who may not understand the why behind my caring for _____ but help them to see You in my caregiving. Please continue to give me the courage to do what is right, no matter the pushback. In Jesus' Name, I pray, Amen.

GETTING THROUGH THE SENSE OF FEELING FORGOTTEN

> "God alienated my family from me; everyone who knows me avoids me. My relatives and friends have all left."
> Job 19:13-14 (The Message)

As I have mentioned, this season will challenge you on so many levels. And one of those levels is your feeling of loneliness and being forgotten or left behind. Job also experienced this sense, and we see where he identified God as the Person who orchestrated the events that resulted in his sense of loss. Is that what you feel today? It's God's fault? It is ok to admit it out loud because once you can admit it, you can begin to move past it and see that it isn't God's fault. It is, however, something God has allowed you to go through. Perhaps it helps you see Him clearly, gain a closer relationship with Him, learn how to lean on Him and trust Him, and change your perception of the event that led you to care for your loved one from tragedy to a witness of God's goodness.

Yes, I know that it is hard; it was hard for me. Friends don't seem to know quite what to say, or they either assume you are too busy, and most times you will be, so they stop inviting you to events or continue to expect you to operate as you did before becoming a caregiver! All as you struggle with how to care for your loved one and care for yourself.

I do believe that God isolates us so we can truly see where our faith is and what we think about Him. Is He the God of the universe, the God who created you in His image, the God who does genuinely love you and will make way for you? All of this gets ironed out in your time of isolation. Embrace it, it will only last as long as it takes you to honestly understand who God is genuinely.

REFLECTIONS:

- Are you blaming God for this season?
- Are you willing to embrace this time of isolation, dig deep, and discover what you believe about God?
- Talk with your heavenly Father (confess what is on your heart).

I AM WITH YOU

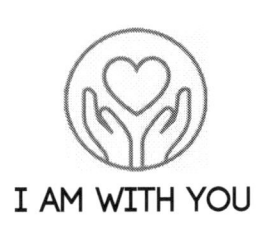

"And I will ask the Father, and he will give you another advocate to help you and be with you forever—the Spirit of truth. The world cannot accept him, because it neither sees him nor knows him. But you know him, for he lives with you and will be in you. I will not leave you as orphans; I will come to you. Before long, the world will not see me anymore, but you will see me. Because I live, you also will live. On that day you will realize that I am in my Father, and you are in me, and I am in you." John 14:16-20 (NIV)

Feeling alone in this season is expected. Although you will encounter other caregivers who can lend comfort through shared experiences and similarities in caregiving, no one can truly understand how you feel and what you are going through. Caregiving is a special and unique call I believe God only gives to those He knows He can trust. That's YOU! I can hear you; you're thinking, "I wish He didn't trust me so much!" It's the exact thing I thought and said when I first became my mother's caregiver. You know that God has a PERFECT plan for your life and the life of your loved one. However, His definition of "perfect" isn't like ours, and that's where the rub comes in. We as humans want and wish everything to be nice and easy; that's perfect for us, and if we are honest, each of us has a version of what is easy and pleasant. So "perfect" varies from person to person. Not so with our God. He has a definition we don't know or understand as it plays out in our lives. Remember, you walk by FAITH, and your faith in Him will help you accept His will and His definition of perfect for your life.

Please know that He has not left you alone nor forgotten you. He has given you a part of Him that will comfort and guide you throughout this season. The Holy Spirit is in you, so cultivate a relationship with Him and allow Him to reveal how much God loves you. Allow Him to comfort you when you feel you are the only person in the world experiencing this season. The Holy Spirit will bring words of comfort to you through scriptures and other individuals that will speak to your unique situation. He will bring songs to your mind that will give you joy and put a smile on your face. Trust God and tune your ear to the Holy Spirit.

ACTION STEPS:

- The Holy Spirit is the third part of the Trinity. He is the Person of God who has taken up residence in your heart. He has a very specific role in your life. He has been called the Helper, the Comforter, the Intercessor, and the Counselor. All of these Names identify how the Holy Spirit works in your life. Stop and ask the Holy Spirit to comfort you when you feel lonely.

PRAYER:

Dear Lord, I know Your word says that Your Holy Spirit lives in me, and I believe Your word. I come asking for the Holy Spirit to provide me with comfort today. I feel alone in this season of caregiving, and I need to know that You are here with me. I'm asking for a hug from You today, Lord. Holy Spirit, please provide comfort and guide me toward the truth of who You are in my life and who I am as a child of God. In Jesus' Name, Amen.

ALLOW GOD TO GUIDE YOU

"The Lord will guide you always; he will satisfy your needs in a sun-scorched land and will strengthen your frame. You will be like a well-watered garden, like a spring whose waters never fail."
Isaiah 58:11 (NIV)

As you embark upon your journey as a caregiver, often depending on the illness, you may not know how long the journey will last. In the beginning, it will seem unbearable that there will be so many competing voices of advice and well-intentioned "help." However, the help and concerned voices stop somewhere along the way, and they move on, but you are still there, caring for your loved one. Whom do you turn to, and where do you find advice and wisdom you KNOW you can trust? The answer is simple, God! He is your North Star. Making time for Him, for you to be in His presence, will provide the space you need to hear Him speaking to you, words of comfort, peace, and direction on the way forward. Seek Him and Trust Him!

ACTION STEPS:

- Set aside a particular time of the day or week to be in His presence to create some alone time with God. In that time, worship Him, sing praise to Him, and tell Him how much you appreciate all He has done for you. Then sit and listen. Now there will be times when you will not hear anything, and that's ok because you will feel His peace. Other times you will receive guidance. It can solve a problem or a sudden urge to contact someone. All of this is God speaking to you. Listen and then do.

GOD IS STANDING WITH YOU

"No one will be able to stand against you as long as you live. I will be with you, just as I was with Moses. I will not leave you or abandon you." Joshua 1:5 (CSB)

There are days when you feel invincible, and then there are the other 363 days of the year when you don't!! Life is hard, and sometimes it gets harder before it gets easier! Caregiving adds more to an already overfull plate! However, living the life that God has called you to is never supposed to be easy; it is supposed to challenge you and move you toward a closer relationship and reliance on Him. And trust me, caregiving will force you to RUN to God for assistance.

The scripture today highlights Joshua taking the leadership role from Moses. He had HUGE shoes, well maybe sandals, to fill. Can you imagine how scared he must have felt, witnessing all that God had done through Moses? Now let's turn the focus from Joshua to you. Your mountain of caregiving is huge, and looking at it, you may believe there is no way you could ever climb it. But you can and you will with God's help. He is right beside you and will not leave or abandon you.

REFLECTIONS:

- Meditate on today's scripture. Just as God was with Moses, Joshua, David, Paul, etc., He is with YOU. God is no respecter of persons, so take courage and remind yourself that God is right there with you.
- Talk to the Father (tell Him how much you need and appreciate His presence).

YOU HAVE BEEN CHOSEN

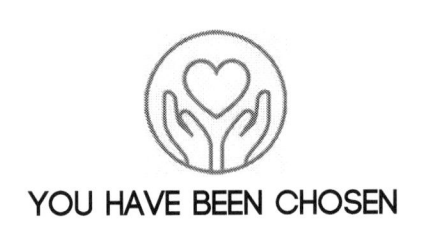

> "So, chosen by God for this new life of love, dress in the wardrobe God picked out for you: compassion, kindness, humility, quiet strength, discipline. Be even-tempered, content with second place, quick to forgive an offense. Forgive as quickly and completely as the Master forgave you. And regardless of what else you put on, wear love. It's your basic, all-purpose garment. Never be without it." Colossians 3:12-14 (The Message)

Please do not believe for a minute that you are alone. In fact, the opposite is true. You have the One Person who matters the most on your side. That is God, and today you see that He has chosen YOU. He chose you not to live a life of frustration, dread, and loneliness but a new life where you get to manifest His qualities and attributes to your loved one whom you care for and the world. Yes, my friend, you have a world ministry!

I don't want to scare you or add more to your already full plate. I want to impress upon you today that God has chosen YOU. He loves you and has given you His character that will allow you to continue with this season in your life.

Today focus on your relationship with Him and how to be more like Him.

You have been chosen!

ACTION STEPS:

- Take a good look at how you have been caring for your loved one. Does it reflect the character of God? Do you exhibit compassion, kindness, humility, etc., as referenced in today's scripture?
- Identify those areas where you can be more like God and ask Him to help you.
- Talk with your heavenly Father.

WHOM ARE YOU LOOKING TO FOR HELP

"God is our refuge and strength, an ever-present help in trouble."
Psalm 46:1 (NIV)

As you learn to master this season of caregiving, it is essential for you to realize that you will need help. However, it is equally important that you know where to seek help. Loneliness can cause you to seek help from the wrong people as you are desperate for companionship or encouragement. However, our scripture teaches that God is the first Person from whom you seek help, guidance, assurance, and revelation. He is YOUR refuge. A refuge is a place you go when you're in trouble that provides safety. This may come as a surprise to you, but you're in trouble all the time. There will be no point in your life when you will not need help from God. Even on your GREAT days, you still need God, and He will be there too.

So, who are you looking for or running to for assistance? Is it God, or do you run to social media and see what the "experts" say? Do you call your best friends or the doctor? All of these are ok once you have consulted with God first! He is the One you are to run to first. He is the One who will provide you with His strength to master the day and all of its trials and tasks—God and God alone. Seek Him first!

ACTION STEPS:

- Today I want you to actively say out loud: "Today, I will seek the Lord and His help." Do not make a decision without first actively asking God for clarity and revelation.
- Talk to the Father (tell Him how you will seek Him today and how thankful you are for the privilege of being in relationship and fellowship with Him).

YOU ARE NOT FORGOTTEN

"Zion says, 'The Lord has abandoned me; the Lord has forgotten me!' 'Can a woman forget her nursing child, or lack compassion for the child of her womb? Even if these forget, yet I will not forget you. Look, I have inscribed you on the palms of my hands; your walls are continually before me...'" Isaiah 49:14-16 (CSB)

Being alone and feeling alone are two distinct concepts or ideas. Being alone, one could argue, is physical; you are alone in a room or house. However, the second is a feeling, an emotion, and we know that emotions can be misleading. I want to concentrate on "being" alone for a moment. You are a being created by the Being God. The mere existence of your being suggests that you are not alone but that you exist because of Him. You are a follower of The Great Being, and God knows you cannot live without Him. Today's scripture shows just how much He is truly connected to YOU...His created being! God is telling the children of Israel that He would and could never forget them. You, too, have been grafted into the kinship of Israel through the shed blood of Jesus...therefore God has not nor will He ever forget you!

You may feel alone but KNOW within your heart that you will never BE alone! Do not allow the enemy to suggest that you are alone and no one cares. God cares and is always with you. I mean, how can He forget you? He's got your name tattooed on His hand!!!

REFLECTIONS:

- Am I lonely?
- Have I in any way fostered this sense of loneliness by isolating myself from friends and family?
- Do I really believe and know that God is always with me?

ACTION STEPS:

- Read today's scripture throughout the day. Think about it. How does it make you feel? Does it give you a new sense of how much God values you?
- Reconnect with family or friends that will encourage and support you.

THE CONTINUAL PRESENCE OF GOD

"Where can I go to escape your Spirit? Where can I flee from your presence? If I go up to heaven, you are there; if I make my bed in Sheol, you are there. If I fly on the wings of the dawn and settle down on the western horizon, even there your hand will lead me; your right hand will hold on to me." Psalm 139:7-10 (CSB)

There is no place you can go where God is not there! This is to provide comfort to you!! No matter where you find yourself...God is there with you. So, let's look at loneliness through God's lens. Of course, He isn't alone; He is three in one. He created all the earth and Us for fellowship. So, when He sees His creation (YOU) crying and moping about, what do you think He thinks?

Let's look back to Genesis when Cain is angry with Able. God seeks him out and asks, "Why are you angry." I imagine God asking you, "Why are you lonely?" He asks the question not because He does not know but for you to admit and recognize where you are. Perhaps you have bought into the lies of the enemy that consistently tell you that you are alone; that no one else has EVER gone through this; that your issue is unique, one of a kind...which probably isn't the case, but even if that were true, so what! God is with you!

In this psalm, David tells you that you can't go anywhere God is not!!! NOWHERE. Even though He created you and broke the mold, your season of caregiving will not break you because He is there right with you to guide you, comfort you, and be your ever-present help in a time of need. Caregiving definitely fits into that category. A time of need!

REFLECTIONS:

- Am I lonely?
- Have I in any way fostered this sense of loneliness by isolating myself from friends and family?
- Do I really believe and know that God is always with me?

ACTION STEPS:

- Read today's scripture throughout the day. Think about it. How does it make you feel? Does it give you a new sense of how much God values you?
- Reconnect with family or friends that will encourage and support you.

SUBMITTING TO GOD

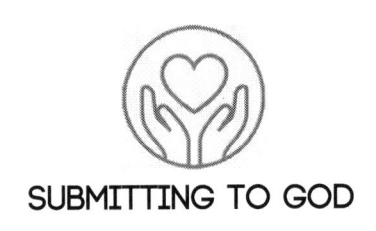

"So let God work his will in you. Yell a loud no to the Devil and watch him scamper. Say a quiet yes to God and he'll be there in no time." James 4:7-8a (The Message)

Submitting to God can be challenging at first. Your will is strong; it wants to do what it wants. However, now that you have given your life to Christ, your strong will must bow before the Lord and allow His Spirit to guide you, especially now that you have been given the added responsibility of caregiving. It isn't that you stop being you, but you pause and ask God if what you are about to do or want to do is okay with Him. You pause and wait. This was something I had to learn; my personality is to get out and do, but as I grew, I had to learn this; my nature is to get out and do this, but as I grew closer in my relationship with God...no objection or silence. Then I moved forward. There have been times when His voice was loud and clear that I was not supposed to be going in the direction I was in. Other times He allowed me to start in a direction but then revealed another way. The lesson is, ask FIRST!

REFLECTIONS:

- Are you submitting your day to God?
- Are you actively seeking His will for your day and life?
- Talk to your heavenly Father (submit your plans to God and give Him the final approval).

YOUR FAITH WILL BRING YOU COMFORT

> "I recall your sincere faith that first lived in your grandmother Lois and in your mother Eunice and now, I am convinced, is in you also. Therefore, I remind you to rekindle the gift of God that is in you through the laying on of my hands."
> 2 Timothy 1:5-6 (CSB)

Did you know that you have a gift from God? Well, you do; every believer is enabled with certain gifts; spiritual gifts that are to be used for the uplifting of the body as well as gifts that are to be used to bring unbelievers to Jesus, and then some equip us to live our best lives in honor of our Creator. You have the "gift" of caregiving. How do I know this? It is because God has called you into this season of caring for your loved one. He doesn't ask us to do anything He hasn't already equipped us for. So, I want you to dig deep and rekindle your faith. You do this by remembering all the wonderful things God has done for you and brought you through thus far. You count your blessings, you look for the good, and in doing so, you find God.

You exercise your faith to move forward, placing your complete trust in God and KNOWING that He will bring you through. I don't know whether you come from a faith-filled family or not. Really, it doesn't matter. What matters is that you have faith the size of a mustard seed, and you can use that faith in God to help you through this season.

ACTION STEPS:

- List all the things God has done for you, outlining how He has brought you through a difficult situation. Use a journal; it will be your visual memorial to the goodness of God in your life. Similar to what God had the Israelites do as He brought them out of Egypt, where they placed rocks at certain events during their journey as a reminder, your journal will serve as a reminder of the goodness of God to you. Read it when you are lonely, sad, angry, and anxious. Read it often.
- Talk with the Father (thank Him for what He has done).

YOU MATTER TO GOD

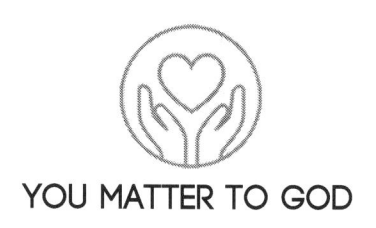

"And my God will meet all your needs according to the riches of his glory in Christ Jesus." Philippians 4:19 (NIV)

Though you may feel lonely during this season, know that you matter to God. Let me say that again, YOU matter to God. He has not left you. He is with you, and your needs not only matter to Him, but He has the solution. The truth is He has already worked out all the issues that continue to nag at you; paying the medical bills, getting caregiving services, employment, etc. All of your concerns, wants, hopes, and needs matter to Him, and He has worked them out for you. He has already outlined every area in your life. Now all you are required to do is follow Him, Trust Him, and Seek Him. God is in the details of YOUR life.

REFLECTIONS:

- When I feel lonely, sad, or overwhelmed, I usually do _____.
- Does what you identified above include going to God?
- If not, I encourage you to seek Him first.
- Talk to the Father (open your heart to God).

REFLECTIONS
ACTION STEPS
PRAYERS

CHAPTER FIVE
Tired or Weariness

Boy, was this huge for me! I was physically drained as well as emotionally. But God, in His infinite wisdom, always provided me with respite and refreshment when I needed it most. And guess what? He will do the same for you!

You'll have many things to do as a caregiver, but that is no excuse to neglect yourself. We often need to remember to take care of ourselves. While pouring all your energy into caregiving and putting you on "the back burner" may seem selfless, it is short-sighted because you run the risk of needing care! Then who will take care of your loved one?

This is why learning to rest is extremely important. Trust God and know that He can and will provide rest. Also, know that it is ok to ask for help. God made us to be a blessing to each other, so look and seek out those who can be a blessing to you during your caregiving season.

I'M JUST TIRED

> "Come to me, all you who are weary and burdened, and I will give you rest." Matthew 11:28 (NIV)

Overcoming the stresses of the days of medication preps, changing linen, perhaps the constant questions that get asked repeatedly or the feelings; whatever your routine consists of, I know it can be exhausting. All you want to do is go somewhere and take a nap! To find some quiet place where no one knows where you are, and you can just be there! To be without the daily routines and responsibilities to enjoy a day where you can actually plan what you want to do.

Those days will come; God will bring people into your life that can ease the burden of caregiving for a time. However, do not forget that He has given you the ultimate responsibility, so you can't abdicate... no matter how much you would like to. Yes, going to God and telling Him you need a break is OK. Understand it is OK to ask your heavenly Father for a reprieve. His word instructs you to go to Him and ask. He will give you the rest you need and deserve!

ACTION STEPS:

- In asking God for rest or help, it is essential that you tell Him precisely what you want. Ask if you want a couple of hours of reprieve or a weekend or week. Ask with the confidence that He is hearing you and with the expectation that He will grant it in His time.
- So, step one, ask.
- Step two, then thank Him in advance of Him answering your prayer.
- Step three, enjoy the day knowing God has heard you and will answer.

ALL I WANT IS TO LIE DOWN

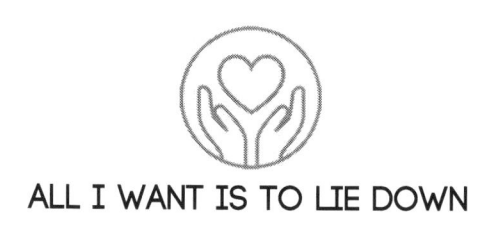

"In peace, I will both lie down and sleep, For You alone, O Lord, make me to dwell in safety." Psalm 4:8 (NASB)

Finding a work-life balance is difficult, but add in caregiving and see what you get. Chaos!!! It's chaos if you don't lay all your goals, priorities, and to-do lists in front of God, asking Him to arrange them. Life is exhausting, and we tend to exhaust ourselves when we think we HAVE to accomplish EVERYTHING every day. Is the fear of missing out or not measuring up to an unrealistic image keeping us on the hamster wheel? No matter the cause, the result is the same, EXHAUSTION!! There are many caregivers, and you are now a part of that calling; how you maneuver it is between you and God.

Your being tired indicates that you have done or are doing too much AND that you are doing it within your own strength and not God's! Since God is your refuge, allow Him to order your life, and listening to the Holy Spirit will make room for you to relax and, yes, GET SOME SLEEP!

REFLECTIONS:

- How often are you tired? Is it more than two times within the week?
- Are you doing too much?
- Do you consistently lay your day, each day before God, as King Solomon advises in Proverbs 16:3?

ACTION STEPS:

- As you talk with God each morning, give Him all the day's priorities and activities. Give Him the full details. Highlight what you think is important, then at the end, ask Him to order your day! As you go about your day, when things aren't going as you have "planned," recall what you asked God to do that morning and rest in knowing that He is in control.

TIRED

> "Truly my soul finds rest in God; my salvation comes from him."
> Psalm 62:1 (NIV)

I admit that I was tired of many things during my caregiving season; tired of the routine of getting up early to give my mother her thyroid medication because that particular medication had to be taken on an empty stomach an hour before eating. So, the days of my sleeping in were gone.

I was tired of the "negotiations" with my mother to get her to cooperate with the day's schedule. I was tired of my endless battles with the Medicare provider and arranging my life around her. Yes, I was tired, but mostly I was tired of being tired! What was my solution? I brought everything to God. In looking back, I see that God not only allowed me to vent and voice my attitudes, but also my need for a break, my need to make a particular conversation with the health insurance rep to generate the desired outcome, and the need for His assurance that I was doing this season in a way that was pleasing to Him and that my mother felt loved. I considered myself a little brat, but God, in His unconditional love for me, allowed it...for a while. As I continued to bring my tiredness to Him, He rearranged my priorities and attitude. And suddenly I realized I wasn't as tired as I had been!

REFLECTIONS:

- The lesson is to learn to bring everything to God and watch how He will meet your needs and transform not only the environment but You to create a less stressful season of caregiving.

DON'T GIVE UP

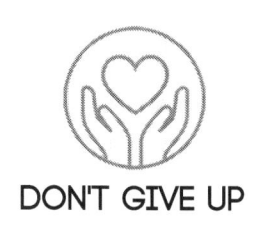

> "But as for you, brethren, do not grow weary of doing good."
> 2 Thessalonians 3:13 (NASB)

It's hard always to do what's right; at least, it is for me sometimes. Learning to be the bigger person when convicted by the Holy Spirit, who corrects our behavior, is a worthwhile process. Surrendering to God allows Him to transform you into a new creature...right? Yet being the one always to concede can be exhausting, and being the one whom everyone turns to for advice and comfort can be time-consuming. This can be hard but not impossible.

God is an excellent God and expects us to follow His example in our Savior, Jesus. Now I know you aren't perfect, but I encourage you to wake up each day to allow the Holy Spirit to guide you so that you will speak and do what is right and pleasing to God.

Today's scripture sends you encouragement to continue; I send encouragement to continue. Do not let your physical and emotional fatigues overshadow who you are. YOU are a child of the Most High God HE created to do Good works!

Your season of caring for your loved one is an outward demonstration of your "good works" being manifested!

ACTION STEPS:

- Write all the ways your life brings honor and glory to God.
- Then close with a prayer of thanksgiving for God using your life to bear witness to His glory.

THIS ISN'T ABOUT YOU

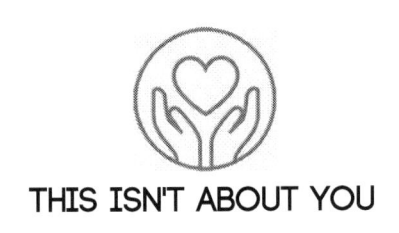

"The one who blesses others is abundantly blessed; those who help others are helped." Proverbs 11:25 (MSG)

Did I mention I'm an only child? Yea, and with that comes a level of self-centeredness that I'm not proud of, but I must be honest. As you know, caring for others and being self-centered does not make for a good mix. Being a caregiver requires, no, it demands that you put your needs aside and put the needs of the person you are caring for first! That was something I had to learn to do. Although I was caring for my mother, whom I loved dearly, I had to address my self-centeredness and allow God to change my focus, and He did.

One beautiful thing about God is that He uses others to bless others. You are a blessing to God; your willingness to bless the person He has given you this season of caregiving blesses God. But it doesn't stop there. He will bless you for your obedience. You aren't supposed to accept because you want to be blessed. You accept His call for this season because you trust Him and desire to be obedient to whatever He calls you to. Because of those reasons, He blesses you because you have answered His call sincerely and with trust.

Yes, you may be tired, but God will continue to bless YOU.

REFLECTIONS:

- Where do you stack on the being self-centered latter?
- Where is your focus during this season? Is it on God and what He wants or on you and what you want?
- Talk with your heavenly Father (ask Him to help you keep Him in focus).

YOUR WEAKNESS, GOD'S PERFECTION

> "But he said to me, 'My grace is sufficient for you, for my power is made perfect in weakness.' Therefore I will boast all the more gladly about my weaknesses, so that Christ's power may rest on me." 2 Corinthians 12:9 (NIV)

God is the ultimate example of getting the most out of everything… including you. Even in your weakness, God uses it to show Himself perfect. How? Because your weakness indicates that you can't do it yourself, you need help, and He is the One to provide the exact help you need.

While I was on active duty, it was amazing, even to me, that I could care for my mother and continue with my career. The days were hard and endless, but because of God, I was able to meet the demands of my job and the demands of caring for my mother. Since God is no respecter of people, what He did for me and through me, He is willing to do for and through you!

Change your perception of your "weakness" from an inability to a partnership with God. You do what you can, and He does what you can't.

ACTION STEPS:

- Do you perceive yourself as weak or unable to manage this caregiving journey? Why or why not?
- List the positives you have as a caregiver.
- List the negatives you have as a caregiver.
- Take both lists and go before the Lord. Celebrate and thank Him for those qualities and areas that are positive; then ask for His help and grace to accomplish what you can't on the negative list.

CALL ON GOD

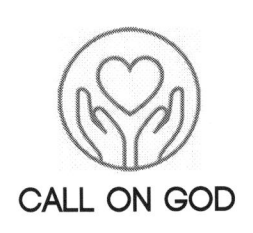

"On the day I called, you answered me; you increased strength within me." Psalm 138:3 (CSB)

As a daughter or son of God, you have direct access to Him. How often do you use this special privilege? Do you go to Him daily, seeking His guidance and help? If the answer is yes, add to your request the need for help in providing rest for your soul, spirit, and body.

If, however, the answer is no, that you don't go to God, then the follow-up question is, WHY NOT? It's another gift He gives you. Today's scripture lets you know that when you call upon the Lord, HE WILL ANSWER YOU. Granted, sometimes the answer we may not want to hear, but He does answer. Our God desires that we go to Him for EVERYTHING. Rest is not off the table! So go to Him and continue to go to Him. Make it a consistent priority for each day of your life.

You will find that as you learn to go to Him, your prayers and requests will turn from being about what you need, which is perfectly acceptable because we all need God's help to go to Him on behalf of those around you: a neighbor, friend, your loved one whom you care for, and others the Holy Spirit will lay on your heart.

Going to God is what He wants. He delights in you spending time with Him. Go to Him and ask Him for rest.

REFLECTIONS:

- When you pray to God, do you expect Him to answer?
- Do you lay out everything that is in your heart, or are there some things you believe you shouldn't bother God with?
- Talk with your heavenly Father (God wants to be in the details of your life, He cares about everything).

THE CHOICE IS UP TO YOU

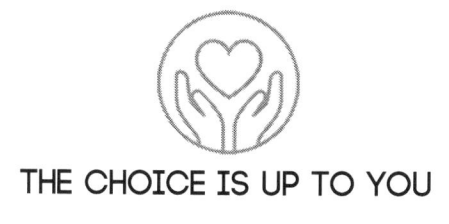

> "The Lord answered her, 'Martha, Martha, you are worried and upset about many things, but one thing is necessary. Mary has made the right choice, and it will not be taken away from her.'"
> Luke 10:41-42 (CSB)

This is a scripture you should be very familiar with. I've heard it preached and taught in many different ways, but today I want to focus on what Jesus says to a frazzled Martha. Jesus acknowledges all that Martha is attempting to do. And really, who can blame her? After all, Jesus is at her house!!! In the gift of hospitality, she wanted Him to feel welcomed. I'm sure a million things needed to be done to do this, but what were those things that HAD to be done?

Being busy has a price, and that is exhaustion and missing out! Martha was missing out on spending quality time with the Messiah!

Caregiving is exhausting and can be overwhelming at times; however, you get to choose between what MUST be done, what NEEDS to get done, and what SHOULD be done. All three categories have a timeframe assigned to them. Could your exhaustion result from not assigning a task to the proper category?

REFLECTIONS:

- What have you neglected because of your busyness?
- Have you assigned your daily tasks to the proper category? A relook may show where you can rearrange tasks and delegate them to someone else. The ultimate goal is to carve out some time for you to rest.
- Talk with your heavenly Father (ask Him to show you where you can do the reshuffling of tasks).

FINDING CONTENTMENT

"I've learned by now to be quite content whatever my circumstances. I'm just as happy with little as with much, with much as with little. I've found the recipe for being happy whether full or hungry, hands full or hands empty. Whatever I have, wherever I am, I can make it through anything in the One who makes me who I am." Philippians 4:11-13 (MSG)

Learning to be content in this season of caregiving is the key to how well you adjust. This new season may have thrown you for a loop... initially, but as you have settled into your season of caregiving, you have begun to get your stride...right? In a sense, getting your stride of the daily routines and requirements is learning to be content with where you are right now.

We know everything has its time with God, so this season will not be permanent. There will come a time when it will be over. Your role is to learn the secret to being content. And that secret is putting your faith in Jesus, learning to trust Him daily to help and equip you throughout this and other seasons.

REFLECTIONS:

- Looking back to when you first began your role as a caregiver, do you see a difference in yourself?
- Have you developed a routine?
- Do you have content with where you are?
- Talk to the Father (giving God praise for bringing you this far and faith to continue to the end).

COUNTING ON GOD

> "Counting on God's Rule to prevail, I take heart and gain strength. I run like a deer. I feel like I'm king of the mountain!"
> Habakkuk 3:19 (MSG)

Caregiving can be a unique opportunity for you as the caregiver to focus on your relationship with God. After all, without Him, the season will be more difficult, and your level of frustration and exhaustion will soar to new highs. Yet, if you focus on Him and your relationship with Him and see that caregiving is a tool He uses to work THROUGH you, the journey becomes something altogether different.

Walking with the Lord during this time means that you are counting on Him, relying on Him to guide you through, open doors of opportunity, and close those doors that will not benefit you or your loved one. Counting on God means you can let go of the heavy load you may feel in shouldering the burden of this season. Why? Because God is the One who is carrying the load. You do all you can and rely on God for the rest of the heavy lifting. God is trustworthy, and putting your trust in Him will never be wrong. Counting on God is the best decision you will ever make!

REFLECTIONS:

- How do you view your role as a caregiver?
- Has your view changed over time?
- What does caregiving mean to you?

REFRESHED

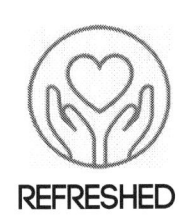

> "I will refresh the weary and satisfy the faint."
> Jeremiah 31:25 (NIV)

What does it mean to be refreshed? When you think of refreshment, what comes to mind? For me, I see a new beginning or a clean slate. All of yesterday's troubles are behind me, and I have a fresh start! The monotony of caregiving can be draining. The much-needed routine for your loved one can limit what you'd like to do.

Yet God! He offers YOU refreshment—a much-needed breath of fresh air. Because God is Lord of the universe, only He knows how and when He will refresh you but know that He will. Your God isn't a man who would lie. If it's in His word, then you can count it as done.

REFLECTIONS:

- What does refresh or refreshment mean to you?
- What are some ways you would like to be refreshed?
- Talk with your heavenly Father (praise Him for being God and thank Him for the refreshment He is bringing to you).

FEASTING ON GOD

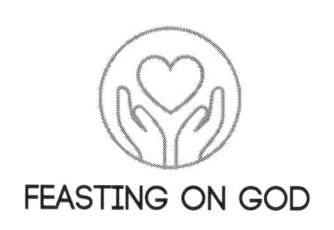

> "My body and my mind may become weak, but God is my strength. He is mine forever." Psalm 73:26 (NCV)

Your body is made of flesh and blood; there is a certain rhythm that you must keep to ensure it maintains optimal performance. Get a good night's rest, diet, exercise, drink plenty of water, AND spend time with your Creator. All of this will ensure optimal performance. You are intricately woven together, and God wants you to maintain what He has given you; after all, you are His temple!

What are you doing to keep yourself healthy? Caregiving is no time to stop caring for yourself and your loved one. Yes, it's hard, but not impossible. God looks at you as a priority just as you look at caring for your loved one as a priority. As you prioritize your loved one, you also must prioritize yourself. It sounds crazy, but it isn't. How can you fully care for your loved one if you're run down with low energy? You can't!

God is your strength, and He has given you the ability to make sound decisions. Learn to make good decisions during this season that will allow you and your loved one to be well taken care of.

PRAYER:

Dear Lord, I am tired and think I may be doing too much. I haven't taken care of Your temple, and I'm asking for You to open up a time in my schedule when I can focus on myself. It sounds selfish to say that out loud, but I need time. I want time to exercise, whether going for a walk or the gym. Please help me make good choices in my diet, my friends, what I watch on TV, and how to prioritize spending time with You. You are my strength, and the closer I get to You, the better I am. In Jesus' Name, I pray, Amen.

GOING DIRECTLY TO THE SOURCE

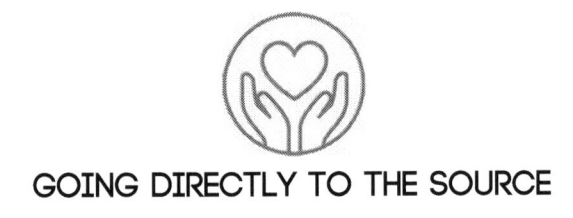

> "Therefore let us draw near with confidence to the throne of grace, so that we may receive mercy and find grace to help in time of need." Hebrews 4:16 (NASB)

Grace and Mercy are your greatest needs during this season. Mercy, because you will have times when you just aren't sure what needs to be done, or the day you're walking in the flesh and not the fruit of the Spirit. You'll need God's mercy that allows you to have missteps. In addition, you will need God's grace as you nurture and mature in the role of caregiver.

Your time of need is now and always. Think about it, is there ever a time when you will not need help from the Lord? No, you'll need Him every day. So, exercise your right as a believer in the Lord; the right to go boldly to Him and speak with Him about your needs—asking for His grace and mercy.

REFLECTIONS:

- Would you say you are a confident person? Do you know who you are in Christ? If the answers are different, it suggests that you haven't answered the second question truthfully.
- Suppose you answered yes to question 1. Where do you get your confidence from? When did you gain this confidence?
- If you answered no to question one, I want you to list everything you know about God—all His characteristics. Then I want you to list what you know He has given you.
- Once you truly know Christ and who you are to Him, you will realize you have His confidence.

MOSES AS AN EXAMPLE OF CAREGIVING

> "The Lord replied, 'I will personally go with you, Moses, and I will give you rest—everything will be fine for you.'"
> Exodus 33:14 (NLT)

Moses had a hard job!! He led the children of Israel out of slavery and started them on their way to becoming a mighty nation. If you've read the Old Testament, you know the Israelites weren't the most cooperative group!! They were needy, forgetful, and whinny, and they brought that to Moses! Occasionally, Moses would go before the Lord on behalf of the people. Several times, he questioned God and asked why HE chose him! Yet we see in Moses a man committed to God and his purpose and role. No matter how angry he got with the people, his first and only action was to go to God. He went to God on everything, and God supplied the response.
There is no other relationship in the Bible, besides Jesus, where we see this intimate relationship between God and man. God was with Moses, and Moses knew and trusted God.

Dear one, God is also with YOU, and even though you may not talk with God as Moses did, which was face-to-face, you can speak to God and expect Him to answer. As with Moses and the children of Israel, God is committed to seeing you through this season, and 'everything will be fine.'

ACTION STEPS:

- Research Moses' relationship with God; it's a beautiful example of how flawed we are and how committed to US God is!

SURROUND YOURSELF IN GOD'S LOVINGKINDNESS

> "'...For the mountains may be removed and the hills may shake, But My lovingkindness will not be removed from you, And My covenant of peace will not be shaken,' Says the Lord who has compassion on you." Isaiah 54:10 (NASB)

When I'm tired, it is not only a physical need to relax but also an emotional one. I need to know that someone cares about me! When you spend your days caring for others, it makes you feel as if no one cares about you! Today I want you to know that someone cares for you. Actually, it is the only Person that really counts...God cares for you. He says so here! His lovingkindness is with you and will always be with you!

As you cobble some much-needed time alone, please allow yourself to meditate on the fact that YOUR Heavenly Father has Love and Kindness toward YOU. Relax, and allow Him to whisper just how precious you are to HIM; then, once you have, allow Him to refresh your spirit and get back in the ring of life!

REFLECTIONS:

- What do you do for yourself that helps refresh you?
- How often do you do something just for you that brings you joy and relaxation? If you do not, please start!
- Express yourself to your Father.

STRENGTH FROM GOD

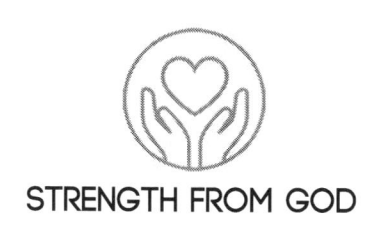

"The Lord is my strength and my shield; my heart trusts in him, and he helps me. My heart leaps for joy, and with my song I praise him." Psalm 28:7 (NIV)

Dear one, today I'd like you to focus on why God provides you with His strength. It's because YOU have placed your trust in Him. By trusting Him, you have given Him full access to help you in this time of need. As a caregiver, there are days, probably like today, when you are exhausted from caring for your loved one. This isn't to say you don't love your loved one; you're tired! Yet, you recognize that this journey is a journey you must go through, and hopefully, you also realize that this is a journey you must go through. This need isn't just to provide care to your loved one but also for YOU. This is a chance God uses to show you who He is and all He has placed in you! Trust me; you have so many gifts, talents, and, yes, strength inside of little ole you!

Continue to Trust Him and praise Him for all that He has and will do!

PRAYER:

Dear Lord, I'm tired!! I need a day or a couple of hours to myself. I ask that You help me to allow You to work in me. Please help me to take one day at a time with You and in You. I put my complete trust in You today, and I ask that You give me all that I need this day to bring You honor and glory. I praise You, God, because You are worthy. And it is my prayer that this season of caregiving grows me closer to You and my loved one.

SOAR LIKE AN EAGLE

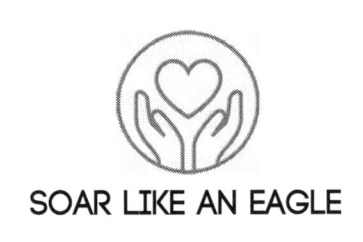

> "He gives power to the tired and worn out, and strength to the weak. Even the youths shall be exhausted, and the young men will all give up. But they that wait upon the Lord shall renew their strength. They shall mount up with wings like eagles; they shall run and not be weary; they shall walk and not faint."
> Isaiah 40:29-31 (TLB)

God is a giving God; He is generous to His children; all you need to do is ask. The Bible declares that we can ask Him for our heart's desires, and IF it is per His will for you, He will grant it. Some things are always in His will for you: wisdom, peace, assurance, fellowship with Him, and strength. All His children can ask for these every day of the week and know that He will provide.

What are you in need of today? Is it strength to tackle the challenges of the day, wisdom to make the right decisions for yourself and your loved one, and assurance that He is with you and the outcome will be by His will?

Go to God, lay down your burdens, allow His magnificent strength to engulf you, and see how high you fly!

REFLECTIONS:

- What are you in NEED of, not what you want, but need? Often, we focus on the outside and "things." This time, concentrate on what you need to make YOU a better caregiver and grow closer to the Lord.

ACTION STEPS:

- Surrender to a prayer of thanksgiving to the Lord for His generosity!

REFLECTIONS
ACTION STEPS
PRAYERS

CHAPTER SIX
Sorrow

Sorrow can accompany other feelings, such as grief and loneliness: the sadness of coming to the realization of what is versus what was supposed to have been; the dreams that will not materialize, that is what can bring on sorrow the most - remembering the plans you had. Perhaps if you are caring for a child with a disability, the sorrow may be in them not growing up to be the man or woman you have envisioned.

Yes, sorrow comes when we come face to face with reality. It also comes as you witness the struggle and perhaps suffering that your loved one experiences. It will be hard, but as with all the other emotions you will experience during your caregiving season… CONTINUE TO TRUST GOD!

A TROUBLED HEART

> "Don't let your hearts be troubled. Trust in God, and trust also in me." John 14:1 (NLT)

What a wonderful simple command: trust in God and also trust in Christ. Why is it so vital that you place your trust in Him? Simply because He loves you and has an excellent plan for you. Your circumstances do not reflect God's plan, only a mere snapshot in time. Do not let a snapshot cloud your view of God or His peaceful, prospering plan for you and your loved one. Release the anxiety of trying to figure it all out and learn to trust in God. Learning to trust God is an act of both obedience and will. As you trust Him, you become more and more obedient to His will, but it is a choice, and YOU must choose to trust Him.

REFLECTIONS:

- Are you anxious and nervous about this season of caring for your loved one?
- Can you get a good night's rest, or are you trying to figure things out?

PRAYER:

Dear Lord, help me to trust You. I know I may have tried to do this myself, but now I am weary, scared, and sad about my life. Help me stop focusing on what I do not have or will not be, and help me to focus on You and what I do have. Help me to realize that You are always with me, that You have provided a way for me to be a caregiver, and that I can put my complete trust in You. Help me to relinquish any bitterness I may have toward the person I am caring for, and help me to stop blaming others, whether it be me blaming You, my loved one, me, or someone else. Please help me to focus on trusting You and caring for my loved ones. In return, Lord, I surrender the outcome to You. Amen.

ARE YOU CRUSHED IN SPIRIT

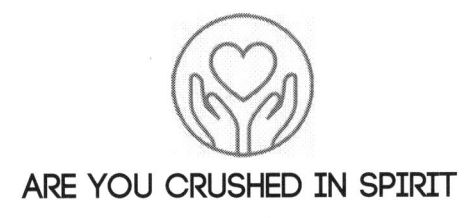

"The righteous cry out, and the Lord hears them; he delivers them from all their troubles. The Lord is close to the brokenhearted and saves those who are crushed in spirit." Psalm 34:17-18 (NIV)

Have you been praying and praying about this season in your life? Perhaps asking God to change the situation...make it go away? At some point in everyone's life, we've all prayed for something to "go away," and when it doesn't happen, what is the next step? It is to continue to pray and trust the Lord.

When we think of God delivering us from our troubles, we think they are to go away, and everything becomes as it was. Unfortunately, that isn't how God views delivering them from their problems. Often the trouble stays, but it is us...YOU that He changes so that the situations no longer take center stage. That is the deliverance!

During this time, God is closer to you than ever before. God experienced the sorrow and brokenness of being separated from His Son, who bore your sins, as the Son being separated from the Father. Yet that did not stop Jesus; He continued to fulfill the prize; you are being reconciled through Him to the Father. This is what He asked of You to continue through; trust Him and know He is close to you and there for you through this time.

PRAYER:

Dear Lord, help me to always look to You for assistance. I confess that my heart is broken and I long for things to be different than they are. I want my old life back, yet I ask Father that You help me to know that this new place You have allowed me to be in can be a place of growth. Please help me to stop focusing on what I don't have and focus on what I do have. Please help me in this role of caregiver. Please give me the tools to be a loving, compassionate caregiver. Give me the assistance to help me bear this new responsibility. Thank You in advance for the help You are sending me and for growth in my relationship with my loved one and You. Amen.

A BROKEN HEART

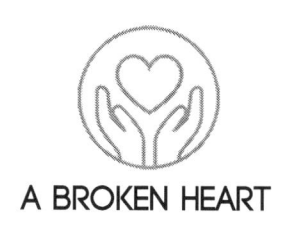

> "He heals the brokenhearted and bandages their wounds."
> Psalm 147:3 (CSB)

Dear one, I know your heart is broken; broken because you witnessed the physical brokenness of your loved one. Yes, I know firsthand how a disease or accident can render the person you knew into the person you're caring for now, who may be slightly or drastically different from the person you knew before the illness or accident. Yet I encourage you to look deep and see that although the physical body of your loved one is broken or their mind may be deteriorating, they are still the person whom you love and who still loves you. Yes, it's hard to witness day in and day out the advancement of a disease BUT know that God is with you! He can and will heal your broken heart, but you must allow Him to do it. How is that done? Constant communion with God, being honest about how you feel and knowing that you cannot allow your feelings to control your mood or daily activities. God understands brokenheartedness. He watched His Son die for YOU. He witnessed how a world He loved turned from Him; therefore, your God knows heartache, yet He would do it all again because of YOU!

Allow Him to wrap His arms around you and provide comfort.

ACTION STEPS:

- Crying is good for the soul and body. Find someplace quiet and away from your loved one—a place where they cannot hear you and CRY. Once you get there, let it out. Know that you will have many days where you will NEED to cry, so do so. Cry and pour out your heart to God and then once you are done, wipe your face, trust God, and continue with your day, knowing that He is with you and can make a way for you.

PRAYER:

Dear Lord, I come on behalf of my brother and sister, asking that You provide them with Your peace and comfort. They don't understand why You chose this path for them and their loved ones, but they trust You. I ask that You heal their broken hearts and that they learn to care for their loved ones. Help them to have good memories of the past while also creating fun and great memories now that they can look back and smile. I pray for their protection, health, and peace during this season of caregiving, and through it, I pray that they grow closer to You! In Jesus' Name, I pray, Amen.

Know that you are loved!

HOW CAN I HAVE JOY IN A TIME LIKE THIS

"For his anger endureth but a moment; in his favour is life: weeping may endure for a night, but joy cometh in the morning."
Psalm 30:5 (KJV)

Having joy in the middle of pain and sorrow may seem unimaginable, but it can happen; it depends on your focus and attitude.

First, your focus is to be on God and only Him. This season will require great strength from you, and the only way you can handle it is through the power of the Holy Spirit. You will need to ask for His strength and guidance each day.

Secondly, your attitude directly reflects your trust and faith in God. If you trust Him, you know He hasn't punished you or your loved one. If you trust Him, you know He will help you; if you trust Him, you will allow His grace to permeate your very being. When you walk in His grace, your attitude toward your role as a caregiver reflects more of His role as a caregiver for us. Do not forget that although the person you are caring for may hold the position of a spouse, grandparent, child, or sibling to God, that person is His son or daughter, and He has given YOU the responsibility for caring for His precious child. You can take great joy in knowing that He entrusted them to you.

REFLECTIONS:

- How much weeping have you been doing?
- Is it time to look for the morning?
- Talk with your heavenly Father.

GIVE IT TO GOD

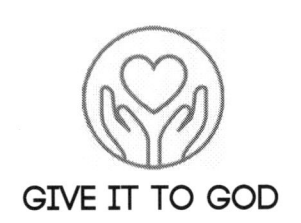

"Cast all your anxiety on him because he cares for you."
1 Peter 5:7 (NIV)

Jesus is not only your Savior but also a Friend who cares for you. It is in His caring for YOU that He offers Himself time and time again to be not just a listening ear but an ear that empathizes with your sorrow and, ultimately, an ear that can fix what troubles you. By going to God and bearing your sorrows holding nothing back, you free yourself of the responsibility of holding everything together (you can't do that anyway). You free yourself from perfection, and you free yourself from feeling alone.

God loves YOU, and as you talk with Him, open your heart and give Him your struggles. It is important to note that YOU must GIVE them to Him. Why? In the giving, you demonstrate your need for Him and trust Him with what you are giving Him, your heart.

REFLECTIONS:

Today reflect on the old Hymn "What a Friend We Have in Jesus."

What a Friend we have in Jesus,
All our sins and griefs to bear!
What a privilege to carry
Everything to God in prayer!
O what peace we often forfeit,
O what needless pain we bear,
All because we do not carry
Everything to God in prayer!

Have we trials and temptations?
Is there trouble anywhere?
We should never be discouraged
Take it to the Lord in prayer!
Can we find a friend so faithful,
Who will all our sorrows share?
Jesus knows our every weakness,
Take it to the Lord in prayer!

Are we weak and heavy-laden,
Cumbered with a load of care?
Precious Savior, still our refuge
Take it to the Lord in prayer!
Do thy friends despise, forsake thee?
Take it to the Lord in prayer!
In His arms He'll take and shield thee,
Thou wilt find a solace there.

STOP LOOKING BACK

> "Do not remember the past events; pay no attention to things of old." Isaiah 43:18 (CSV)

How can you move forward if you consistently are looking back? You can't, so why continue to do so? Taking a survey of your life now and the life of your loved one must be done initially, but you cannot continue to lament what has occurred; recounting the past, perhaps the events that led to this moment, the dreams that are now altered or limited to the freedom you may have now. God is instructing you to STOP! The question is, why? Simply being stuck in the past prevents you from moving forward. God has a plan in all this, and once you accept His will and seek His guidance, you will move forward. Slowly at first, then you'll get your stride, and the next thing you know, you are experiencing a new level of intimacy with God, and the growth you will have made will astonish you. So let go of the past, embrace today, and look forward to tomorrow!

REFLECTIONS:

- What are my thoughts throughout the day? Am I spending my time reliving the events that have led to this moment?
- What do I need that will help me to focus more on today and not what has happened?
- Do I have a group of friends who can help me now?
- Talk with your heavenly Father.

GOD SEES YOU

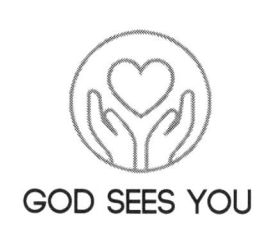

"Lord, my every desire is in front of you; my sighing is not hidden from you." Psalm 38:9 (CSB)

Being disappointed with your current circumstances isn't a sign of weakness but a sign that you're human! You had plans, and now those plans may not be fulfilled; who wouldn't be disappointed? God isn't mad at you for being disappointed or lamenting over this season. Because He is so good, He allows you these outpouring of emotions for a period of time. After which, He expects you to turn your attention to what is in front of you and expectantly wait for His direction.

He knows you; nothing in your life EVER takes Him by surprise! HE LOVES YOU and will help you get through this season.

REFLECTIONS:

- What am I most sorrowful for?
- How long have I been in a state of disappointment? Could it be time for me to turn my attention to God?
- Talk with your heavenly Father.

ACCEPTING GOD'S PEACE

"Peace I leave with you; My peace I give to you; not as the world gives do I give to you. Do not let your heart be troubled, nor let it be fearful." John 14:27 (NASB)

Have you ever really experienced true peace? For many of us, the answer is no, but the question is, why, especially if you are a child of God? Why do we, as believers, not have the peace that Christ has stated He gives us? Could it be that we haven't accepted it? Have you accepted His peace?

How do you find peace in a world where sin seems to be rewarded and "good" people are punished? How do you learn to look past all you see, past the circumstances, perhaps the medical bills, and zero in on Christ? That is how you will find true peace! Focusing on God, reading His word, engaging in private and corporate worship, and regularly chatting with your Savior. During this time, you learn to hear His voice, you learn His character, and you, through the Holy Spirit, begin to surrender to Him. It is in the surrendering of self that God infuses you with Him. As you grow closer to Him, you'll learn to trust Him a little more, and it is through you learning to trust in Him that you will experience His peace, knowing that you have placed your trust in the ONE Person who can make a difference.

REFLECTIONS:

- Do I truly trust God?
- Are you at peace with this season in your life and with your circumstances?

ACTION STEPS:

- For the next week, spend time alone with the Lord each morning and talk to Him. At the end of your conversation, say, "Lord, I trust You in every situation in my life." Say this consistently the entire week; by the end of the week, take a mental survey and see if you are not more at peace than you were before. Then make this a common life practice.

SUFFICIENCY IN CHRIST

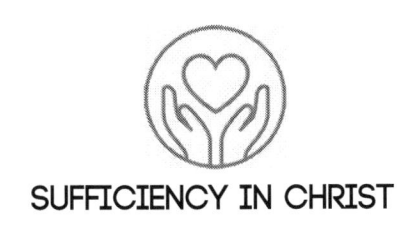

> "But he said to me, 'My grace is sufficient for you, for my power is made perfect in weakness.' Therefore I will boast all the more gladly about my weaknesses, so that Christ's power may rest on me." 2 Corinthians 12:9 (NIV)

God's grace is so amazing! By His grace, you have the ability to not only care for your loved one with joy but to enjoy the season. This season will require everything you've got and more. You will need to ensure your loved one has the best care they need and that you also have the best care you need to continue as a caregiver. As stated earlier and numerous times, this new situation has not surprised God. For His reason, He has allowed this season to come to you, and YOU have the choice of whether you will continue to trust Him and draw nearer to Him or try to do it on your own because you are angry with Him. I recommend trusting Him. He is very near to you and wants to help you during this time; therefore, you must be open and honest with Him about your weaknesses, needs, emotions, and everything else. His grace is more than sufficient, so go ahead and trust Him.

REFLECTIONS:

- Am I trying to do it all myself?
- Have I reached out for help, whether the help is emotional support or respite care?
- Should I be afraid of asking for help?

ACTION STEPS:

- Set aside one hour a day just for you.

KEEP YOUR EYES ON THINGS ETERNAL

"For I consider that the sufferings of this present time are not worthy to be compared with the glory that is to be revealed to us." Romans 8:18 (NASV)

It can be hard not to look at your current circumstance consistently; it is the only thing you can see, right? However, God wants you to walk by faith and not by sight, meaning take your eyes off your current situation and look at God; embrace His promises found in His word and Jesus. Paul challenges you to look beyond your suffering and consider ALL that you gain as a child of God. Notice that this scripture affirms that you will endure suffering. It is inescapable, but once again, it is your attitude during your suffering and hardship seasons where you display your trust and obedience to God.

When you think about all that God has done for you and all that He has planned for you and that one day, you will be reunited with HIM, there is no comparison. This life will be challenging, but with Christ, you look toward the glory that will be revealed in you!

PRAYER:

Dear Lord, I thank You for our relationship, for establishing a relationship with me through Your Son and my Savior Jesus. Thank You for Your love that is unconditional and for Your presence. Lord, I ask that You help me to realign my focus on You. Please help me to allow Your glory to shine through me in this season of caregiving. I love You, Lord. Amen.

TAKE COURAGE FROM GOD

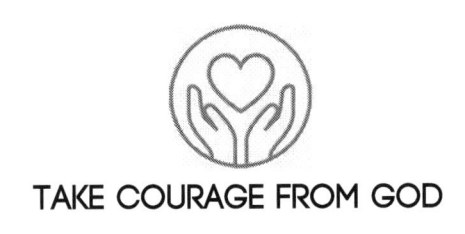

> "These things I have spoken to you, so that in Me you may have peace. In the world you have tribulation, but take courage; I have overcome the world." John 16:33 (NASB)

Jesus had been preparing His disciples for His impending death. Yet we know that it seemed to catch them off guard once it happened. Does your sudden change in life catch you by surprise? Dear heart, know that it hasn't caught God off guard. Jesus challenges us to look at the life He lived here on Earth. He maintained a consistent relationship with the Father; He not only was God personified, but He demonstrated how we live and walk in the fruits of the Spirit. And here in this scripture, He reminds us that because He did it, so can we…YOU. Look to Jesus and His life and follow in His footsteps. His shoes are too big for us to fit into, but just as children try to wear their parents' shoes, God expects us to as well, and while His hands hold you up, you will discover that you are walking with Him!

REFLECTIONS:

- Do I consider myself a worrier?
- Do I want to live a life of peace?
- Is it possible to live a life of peace?
- Am I often anxious about the future?

PRAYER:

Dear Lord, help me just to let things go, fully acknowledging that You have everything under control, to daily come to You for direction, guidance, and help in meeting today's needs and demands. Please help me to learn to take one day at a time with You. Amen.

REST

> "Come to me, all of you who are weary and burdened, and I will give you rest. Take my yoke upon you and learn from me, because I am lowly and humble in heart, and you will find rest for your souls. For my yoke is easy and my burden is light."
> Matthew 11:28-30 (CSB)

Learn how to breathe. We take breathing for granted, but breathing is essential for life. As a caregiver, you must learn to stop among all the chaos and the millions of decisions you must make and breathe. This process forces your lungs to expand and breathe in more, which can be calming. In addition to physically breathing, we must learn to breathe spiritually; to recognize the sabbath. God created and then rested. Your weariness and burdensome feelings come from not allowing your body, mind, and spirit to rest.

In this scripture, God invites you to learn from Him. If He rested, why do you not? Jesus, on several occasions, would go away from the crowds and pray. This was Him breathing and gaining insight from the Father.

Jesus offers His hand to you to allow His grace to fall on you as you learn to breathe; in other words, take one day at a time. It's ok to feel distressed but know that God has already worked out the situation on your behalf.

REFLECTIONS:

- List the thing(s) that you can do that will help you to experience God's rest.

ACTION STEPS:

- Put into action what you listed above.

LEARN TO TRUST GOD

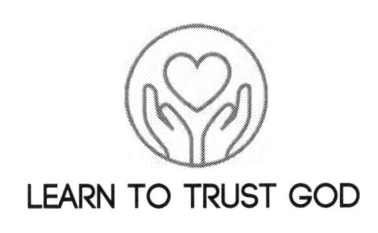

> "The Lord himself goes before you and will be with you; he will never leave you nor forsake you. Do not be afraid; do not be discouraged." Deuteronomy 31:8 (NIV)

Often with sorrow, as you look at the past and remember the good times, you look at your current circumstances and don't see anything good. The future is some mysterious place that, at this point, you may not be able to comprehend or imagine. Everything seems so up in the air and out of your control which can lead to fear of "what's next."

Dear heart, know that God is not only with you every second of the day, but He has already gone into YOUR future and that of your loved one. He has seen it and still encourages YOU not to be afraid. The "what's next" you may not know, but He does, and that you can take comfort in. Just as God was with Joshua and the Hebrew children as they entered the promised land, He is with you. Remember, there were battles and enemies the children of Israel had to fight and conquer to pursue the land God had promised them. You, too, must follow what God has promised you. Stay faithful and remember that He is with you.

REFLECTIONS:

- Am I afraid of the "what's next" in my life?
- Am I truly trusting God in this season?

ACTION STEPS:

- Begin by trusting God with one day. Each morning, wake up, spend time with God, and let Him be in control for THAT day. The next morning, repeat!

CHRIST OUR OVERCOMER

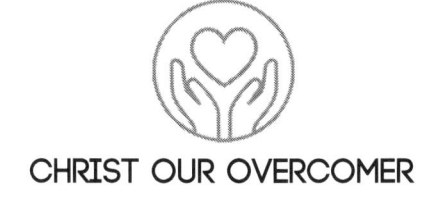

> "These things I have spoken unto you, that in me ye might have peace. In the world ye shall have tribulation: but be of good cheer; I have overcome the world." John 16:33 (KJV)

It can be easy to ask, "Why me or why us?" but the real question is, "Why not you and why not us?" As children of God, we are not immune to hardships. If you think about it, it's during a time of crisis that you grow closer to God, your faith is strengthened, AND those around you see how God is working in your life. You become a living testimony!!!

Jesus tells His disciples that they (we/you) will have hard times. Some things are more complex than others, and each person's experience of hardship will be different. But no one goes through life without experiencing something. Most often, the "something" is unexpected, like caregiving, being laid off from work, a divorce, or a sudden death of a loved one.

I encourage you to remember that Christ has overcome this world. Through Him, He has given you the ability to overcome as you continue to trust Him through your season of caring for your loved one. You too will overcome the feeling of sorrow and soon look at it as God does, an opportunity to grow and show how great a God you serve.

REFLECTIONS:

- How have I adapted to my role as a caregiver?
- How do I feel about this new season in my life?
- Talk to the Father.

THE FORMER THINGS HAVE GONE

> "And God shall wipe away all tears from their eyes; and there shall be no more death, neither sorrow, nor crying, neither shall there be any more pain: for the former things are passed away."
> Revelation 21:4 (KJV)

This season you may find yourself in extreme sorrow as you think of all your plans before you became a caregiver and of the future of your loved one. Sometimes, you must be prepared for their departure to be reunited with Jesus. It's hard and a heavy load to bear. And although going down memory lane can seem helpful in this case, it is not. The enemy can use this as a time to remind you of what you've "missed" or what you will miss, and God wants you to look to Him, allowing Him to show you what you have gained! As with all things, it is crucial for you to keep your dialogue open with God. Go to Him and give Him your sorrow. Allow Him to wipe away your tears. Knowing that it is ok to cry, crying can be very therapeutic. As you release your hurt, sadness, and plans, allow the Holy Spirit to give you new plans to look forward to. Learn to celebrate the little things in life. Letting go of what was, can be challenging, but once you let go of it, you are free to receive the "new" God has in store for you.

REFLECTIONS:

- Am I concentrating too much on what I've lost?
- What are some new things to look forward to?
- How can I take my sorrow and turn it into something positive?
- Talk with your heavenly Father.

REFLECTIONS
ACTION STEPS
PRAYERS

CHAPTER SEVEN

Grief

Now that you have come to the end of your caregiving season, finding peace in the days ahead may be difficult. Yet, God has made provisions for you; He has written a letter of love to you! They are designed to bring you comfort and peace. Your period of mourning is something that you and God must work out. He will give you the time you need to heal, but know that at some point, He will ask that you follow Him and continue with the life He has planned for you.

Know that you are not alone.

DO NOT GRIEVE AS THE WORLD GRIEVES

"Brothers and sisters, we do not want you to be uninformed about those who sleep in death, so that you do not grieve like the rest of mankind, who have no hope. For we believe that Jesus died and rose again, and so we believe that God will bring with Jesus those who have fallen asleep in him. According to the Lord's word, we tell you that we who are still alive, who are left until the coming of the Lord, will certainly not precede those who have fallen asleep. For the Lord himself will come down from heaven, with a loud command, with the voice of the archangel and with the trumpet call of God, and the dead in Christ will rise first. After that, we who are still alive and are left will be caught up together with them in the clouds to meet the Lord in the air. And so we will be with the Lord forever. Therefore encourage one another with these words." 1 Thessalonians 4:13-18 (NIV)

Many distinctions separate us, as Christians, from non-believers, the most important being our reliance on and acceptance of Jesus Christ as Savior, and then another, I believe, is how we grieve the loss of our loved ones, which is what today's scripture defines. We know that we do not die without hope. Our hope is in Jesus, therefore, when we sleep, it is only temporary. Therefore, when we (you) grieve, it's different. We, as Christians, celebrate the lives of our departed family and friends; we memorialize them and acknowledge their impact on our lives and how they made us laugh and cry. We do not mourn with despair but celebrate the homegoing, knowing we will see them again.

REFLECTIONS:

- Take some time today to reflect on who Jesus is, what He means to you, and how knowing Him has changed your perspective and perception of life.

DO YOU KNOW HOW SPECIAL YOU ARE

"For the Lord your God is living among you. He is a mighty savior. He will take delight in you with gladness. With his love, he will calm all your fears. He will rejoice over you with joyful songs." Zephaniah 3:17 (NLT)

Do you really know how special YOU are to God? I mean, really know just how much He loves you? Zephaniah captures just a glimpse of just how much, but this glimpse is so sweet. The Lord, YOUR God, actually sings songs of joy over YOU. He rejoices over YOU! Let that sink in for a moment.

Can you imagine God singing over you as you sleep? I think most of us do not; we just get up and go about our day. The Lord singing over His children just shows how enamored He is with YOU because you are His child. Today's scripture reminds you that God is living with you, which is meant to comfort your soul. The time of loss isn't easy, but it came and will be made easier with God by your side. God lives among YOU, and I encourage you to rest in that knowledge, and then tomorrow morning, before you jump out of bed, be still and silence yourself and hear the songs the Lord sings over you.

REFLECTIONS:

- Really think about how special you are to God.

PRAYER:

Thank God for loving you so much.

BLESSED

"You're blessed when you feel you've lost what is most dear to you. Only then can you be embraced by the One most dear to you." Matthew 5:4 (MSG)

I know it's hard to consider you being blessed at this point in time. Your loved one is now with God, and you may be left with isolation, uncertainty, and grief. However, this scripture encourages you to see your grief as another tool to draw your focus off of yourself and back on God. No one can comfort you like the One who created you. He understands your loss, but He also knows His overall plan for you. Your loved one is now in His presence—no more pain.

As you mourn the loss of your loved one, please do not allow the enemy to trick you into thinking God doesn't love you. He does and wants to provide the peace and comfort only He can. The question is will you let Him?

REFLECTIONS:

- Write how you genuinely feel about the loss of your loved one.

PRAYER:

Pray your letter to God.

REMAIN STEADFAST

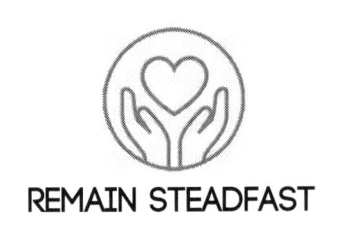

"I remain confident of this: I will see the goodness of the Lord in the land of the living." Psalm 27:13 (NIV)

The loss of your loved one has rocked your world; now, things are unfamiliar and unsettling. A person crucial to you is now gone, leaving a large hole in your heart and life. Will this hole heal? Somewhat, but it will never go completely away, and frankly, you don't want it to. There should remain a little of this to remind you of who that person was to you, don't you think? What will happen is that you will learn to live this life despite the hole; it will grow smaller but not disappear.

How are you to continue with this hole? You continue as a grounded, well-established child of God. You remember who you are and whose you are, recounting the numerous times when God has been there and brought you out of crazy situations, and how He has been there during the great and bad times. You reflect on all that He has done for you during your season of caregiving, and you will proclaim as David has in Psalm 27:13!

REFLECTIONS:

- Do you believe Psalm 27:13? Write down why or why not.
- Where do you place your confidence?
- Do you believe God is good?

PRAYER:

Talk with your heavenly Father.

REMEMBERING GOD'S WORD

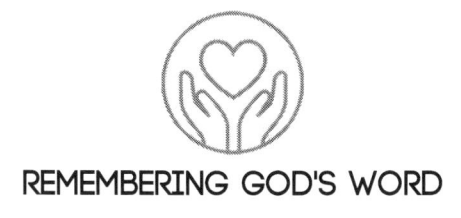

"Remember your word to your servant, for you have given me hope. My comfort in my suffering is this: Your promise preserves my life." Psalm 119:49-50 (NIV)

Now is the time to reflect on God's promises to YOU as His child. If you know anything, should it not be that you can trust God? Trust Him to do exactly what He has said in His word? Today's scripture encourages you to remember who God is and who YOU are to Him, remembering that reflecting on His word will bring you comfort during this time of loss.

ACTION STEPS:

- List some of the scriptures that bring you comfort.
- Now say them out loud, then pray those scriptures to God.

HOPE

> "Having hope will give you courage. You will be protected and will rest in safety." Job 11:18 (NLT)

Psalm 121:2 says that our hope comes from the Lord. This same hope is found in Job, the scripture for today. Hope is a word often used in society and is defined roughly as believing in a better future. It propels one to move forward. However, for Christians, hope is solely based on the Lord Jesus Christ. Jesus is Hope, and having the right relationship with Him means that things will be better; not only do you have a home in eternity, but that RIGHT now, things are being worked out for your good. Therefore, you can rest knowing that Jesus is with you.

Grieving is a multifaceted process experienced differently by the person going through it. Yet for you, a child of the Most High, your hope is anchored in Jesus, and although you miss your loved one, remember where your hope comes from and know that you are loved and not alone.

REFLECTIONS:

- What does hope mean to you?
- Write down how your grieving process has been.
- Do you feel hopeless at times?

PRAYER:

Share your concerns with your heavenly Father.

CALL ON GOD

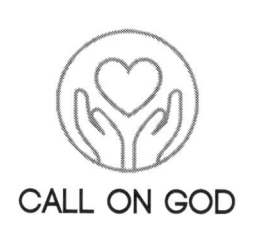

> "Yes, you came at my despairing cry and told me not to fear."
> Lamentations 3:57 (TLB)

I know for me when I experience deep sadness or regret, I tend to stay away from God, surprisingly, just like our relatives Adam and Eve. I try to hide from God's presence because I am too embarrassed by what I have done, or my emotions are so crazy that I don't want to bring that to God! Of course, all of this is contrary to His word, which is clear that He wants and desires that we come to Him with everything, no matter what.

You may be experiencing days when you don't want to get out of bed or want to eat all the ice cream or cake or fill in the blank with what you want. Well, I say do those things, at least for now. But know that one day those impulses must come to an end. But in the midst of all that, GO TO GOD. When you cry out to God, He hears you and wraps His arms around you, and provides you with His peace and love. Do not ever think there could be a time when you cannot go to Him and express whatever is on your mind or in your heart. He is your Creator who loves you as a father and mother. He cares for you!

ACTION STEPS:

- Let it go! Take this time to write down everything that is in your heart.

CRY

"Jesus cried." John 11:35 (NCV)

A friend talks about not crying because she needs "to be strong," and I hate it. Since when did crying become a weakness? Here we see the Savior of the world crying! So, if Jesus can cry, so can you! Being strong is facing your fears and the reality of your situation and moving forward to change the situation if that situation is unpleasant and not in alignment with God's will for you. Being strong does not suppress your emotions to the point where they are bottled up. Studies have shown that when we suppress our feelings, they will find a way to be released, often resulting in health issues!

So, cry hard and as often as you need to. It shows you are human and that you love your loved one.

REFLECTIONS:
- Are you trying to keep up a "good" appearance for others? Why or why not?

ACTION STEPS:
- Find a quiet place or a good friend where you can be you, surrender to your emotions, and let them out. Then take note of how much better you feel and thank God.

IT IS TIME TO MOVE ON

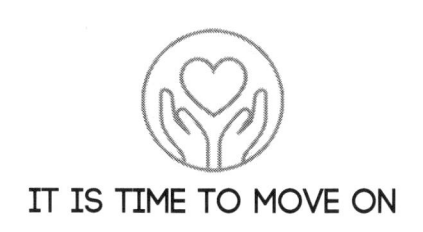

"After the death of Moses the Lord's servant, the Lord spoke to Joshua son of Nun, Moses' assistant. He said, 'Moses my servant is dead. Therefore, the time has come for you to lead these people, the Israelites, across the Jordan River into the land I am giving them.'" Joshua 1:1-2 (NLT)

Dear one, I know that these words may sound harsh or even cruel but know that they are not meant to be. Grieving lasts for a season, but that season must come to an end. Our God leaves nothing to chance. He gives us His words to guide us and lead us toward a closer relationship with Him and instructions for living here on earth. Today you see God telling Joshua, "It's time to move on." They, the children of Israel, had been mourning the death of Moses, and in their mourning, they were not moving forward to their destiny.

Your grieving time is only supposed to stop you momentarily. It gives you time to reflect on the times you spent with your loved one; to ensure "life" issues are completed, wills, bills, burial, etc., and adjust to a new life without your loved one. Granted, this doesn't all happen at once, but after you have completed a significant portion of these, it will be time for you to begin your journey without your loved one but NOT ALONE. God is with you, but He will tell you in His sweet way, "The time has come for you to…"

REFLECTIONS:

- Has your grieving been so prolonged that you have stopped living? Perhaps it is so difficult that you need outside assistance from a trusted friend or even a good Christian counselor. God is with you. Ask Him to help you through this season.

PRAYER:

"Dear Lord, I pray for my sister or brother who is hurting at the loss of their loved one. I ask that You comfort them and let them feel Your sweet arms of protection and assurance. Help them know they can and must continue and that You have given them the strength to do so. If this weight is too heavy to bear, I ask, Lord, that You direct them to someone You have ordained to help them through this process. And in the end, help them to be able to remember their loved one while continuing on the road ahead. It is in Jesus' Name I pray, Amen."

RESTORING YOUR HEART

"The Lord is near to those who have a broken heart. And He saves those who are broken in spirit." Psalm 34:18 (NLV)

Now more than ever, you must know that God is with you. Losing your loved one doesn't mean you are currently on your own; God is with you and will never leave you. As your heart breaks at the thought of your loved one, know that God weeps with you and is right by your side, feeling every emotion with you.

Your loss does not bring Him joy; He does not delight in your sorrow. God had a plan for your loved one, and whether you agree with God's plan or not, it was His plan, and you are to trust Him.

Do not allow this loss to distance yourself from God; now is the time to draw closer. He has been with you through this season and will be with you for the next one. Trust God!

REFLECTIONS:

- Are you angry with God for the passing of your loved one?
- Are you blaming yourself for the loss of your loved one?
- Are you panicked at the loss of your loved one?
- Talk with your heavenly Father (be honest about how you feel, and after you have voiced your feelings, resolve within yourself to continue to trust God).

THE ROCK

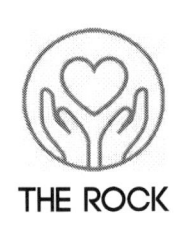

> "The Lord is my rock, my protection, my Savior. My God is my rock. I can run to him for safety. He is my shield and my saving strength, my defender." Psalm 18:2 (NCV)

Today, I'd like you to reflect on God and who He is, and Who you have allowed Him to be to you. The psalmist declares that he has made God his Rock, a formidable structure that keeps him safe and provides shelter and protection. As you continue to mourn the loss of your loved one, you need a Rock. Perhaps your loved ones were your earthly rock providing that safe place for you, your companion or confidant, or the person you shared everything with. Now they are gone, but your heavenly Rock is still with you.

REFLECTIONS:

- Look up the hymn "I Go to the Rock" by Dottie Rambo to sing and ponder.

KNOWING GOD'S HEART

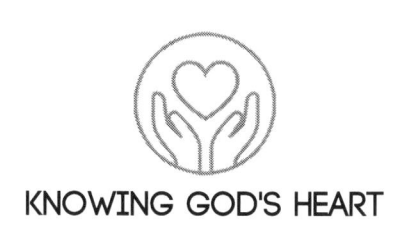

"For the Lord will not turn away from a man forever. For if He causes sorrow, He will have loving-pity because of His great loving-kindness. He does not want to cause trouble or sorrow for the children of men." Lamentations 3:31-33 (NLV)

God is a loving God whose thoughts are far beyond what we can understand. As you mourn the loss of your loved one, it is easy to blame God; after all, He is in control, right? Right, but trying to figure out why He allowed this season in your life and the life of your loved one will zap all the energy and emotion you have...and it's a waste of time!

As a child of God, you come to Him on faith, and that faith is what you need right now to accept the loss; faith that God does know what He is doing and that despite your pain, and perhaps the pain endured by your loved one, God is a loving and caring God.

ACTION STEPS:

- Make a list of all the ways God has shown His mercy and love toward you. Then go to Him in prayer, thank Him for the things on your list, and ask Him to help you through this grieving period.

THE CYCLE OF LIFE

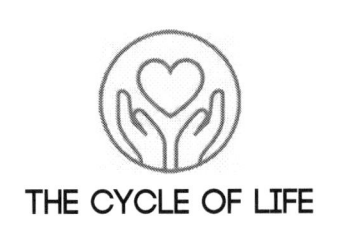

"There is a special time for everything. There is a time for everything that happens under heaven. There is a time to be born, and a time to die; a time to plant, and a time to pick what is planted. There is a time to kill, and a time to heal; a time to break down, and a time to build up. There is a time to cry, and a time to laugh; a time to have sorrow, and a time to dance. There is a time to throw stones, and a time to gather stones; a time to kiss, and a time to turn from kissing. There is a time to try to find, and a time to lose; a time to keep, and a time to throw away. There is a time to tear apart, and a time to sew together; a time to be quiet, and a time to speak. There is a time to love, and a time to hate; a time for war, and a time for peace." Ecclesiastes 3:1-8 (NLV)

Life has a rhythm, and seasons are a part of life's rhythm. I'm sure this scripture is familiar to you, yet we sometimes forget the rhythm of life despite it being all around us; nothing is here forever, nothing. Your loss is significant, and you are allowed to mourn, dear one. Please understand that mourning has an end just as life does. You know this isn't the end and that you will see your loved one again; hence why God does not want you to mourn forever because there will come a time when forever means you being reunited with your loved ones and, most of all, your Savior.

REFLECTIONS:

- This season of caregiving is over. Mourn the loss and with full commitment, move forward to the next season God has for you.
- Share your journey.

WEEPING FOR THE NIGHT

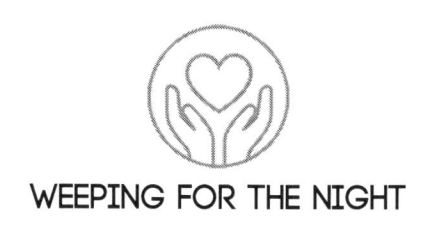

"Oh, sing to him you saints of his; give thanks to his holy name. His anger lasts a moment; his favor lasts for life! Weeping may go on all night, but in the morning there is joy." Psalm 30:4-5 (TLB)

Life is unpredictable even for believers; with this unpredictability, we turn our focus and attention to the One in total control. God does get angry, but His anger isn't directed toward His children. His anger is directed at injustice and inequity. His children received His favor; even when we don't quite understand or feel it, it's there.

Your loss is significant; you must grieve the loss to move forward. Remember, the Lord YOUR God is a forward-moving God, and He will not allow you to stay stagnate. He will allow you time to mourn, and after that time is completed, He will gently instruct you to get up and wash your face (figuratively speaking) and rejoice for the new day is here!

REFLECTIONS:

- Sing to the Lord the hymn "10,000 Reasons [Bless the Lord]" by Matt Redman.

THIS IS ONLY TEMPORARY

"Yet what we suffer now is nothing compared to the glory he will reveal to us later." Romans 8:18 (NLT)

As a believer, it is essential to remember what is important and what things are not so much so. Your loss is significant; however, you must remember that you have a higher priority. As a believer, you are a citizen of Heaven and one day that is where you will be along with your loved one.

Remember that the trials and troubles you encounter now are momentary blips. Your grief will become more manageable, and you can continue. Never forget that life here is temporary, and you have a home in eternity. Trust God and allow His purpose in your life to be fulfilled.

ACTION STEPS:

- Find a quiet space and meditate on God and His word. Ask Him to reveal what He has for you. Be still and listen for His soft voice to discover what God's plan is for you. Talk to your Father and find out what it is.

THIS ISN'T GOODBYE

"You have sorrow now, but I will see you again and then you will rejoice; and no one can rob you of that joy." John 16:22 (TLB)

As you mourn the loss of your loved one here on earth, take comfort in knowing that you will see them again in eternity. Life on earth is temporary and short; some lives are taken earlier than what we deem appropriate, but all things work toward God's purpose. Eternity is forever, where you'll be with your Savior and your loved ones.

Take comfort in knowing you will see them again.

REFLECTIONS:

- Look up the song lyrics for "I'll See You Again" by Westlife to reflect on.

KEEP MOVING FORWARD

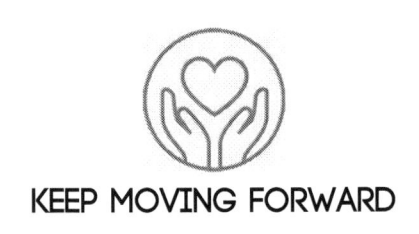

> "And God shall wipe away all tears from their eyes; and there shall be no more death, neither sorrow, nor crying, neither shall there be any more pain: for the former things are passed away."
> Revelation 21:4 (KJV)

Dear one, as you mourn the loss of your loved one, I want to remind you that death isn't the end! It is merely a transition to eternity. There will come a day when not only will you see your loved one again, but all of the pain and suffering that you and others have experienced will be GONE!

As a child of God, remember that this life on earth is temporary, and while you are here, God has a plan and a purpose for you. Keep trusting Him and continue walking the path He has set before you. Cherish the memories of your loved one, live a life that will make them laugh and proud, and above all, live a life that honors and brings glory to God.

ACTION STEPS:

- Do something today that your loved one would enjoy and laugh at.
- Dedicate today to them.

YOU'LL GET THROUGH THIS

"What happiness there is for you who are now hungry, for you are going to be satisfied! What happiness there is for you who weep, for the time will come when you shall laugh with joy!"
Luke 6:21 (TLB)

I know you have been told this probably one hundred times now but I will be the 101st. You will get through this! Everything has its season, and your season of caregiving has come to an end. Yet, there are other seasons ahead of you. Some are great, while others are just ok, and there may be one or two that will be difficult, but in ALL seasons, you, as a child of the Highest God, are to trust God.

It is through His strength and power that you will find joy again, you will be able to laugh again, and you will be able to LIVE again.

ACTION STEPS:

- Do something daily that brings you joy, something just for you.

YOU STILL HAVE A PURPOSE

> "What a wonderful God we have—he is the Father of our Lord Jesus Christ, the source of every mercy, and the one who so wonderfully comforts and strengthens us in our hardships and trials. And why does he do this? So that when others are troubled, needing our sympathy and encouragement, we can pass on to them this same help and comfort God has given us."
> 2 Corinthians 1:3-4 (TLB)

Your God is a BIG picture, God! He sees everything and knows everything. And He knew He could count on you to help others. Your sorrow and anguish will not be senseless; they can and will be used to help others as they, too, experience loss. You then become the one who can provide insight and comfort. Just as others are comforting you now, you will comfort others.

God created us for fellowship: first with Him and then with others. As you continue on your journey and new seasons, this knowledge will be with you, and know that one day God will call upon YOU to encourage and help someone experiencing what you are experiencing now. Nothing is lost in God's economy. He looks after everyone. As He walked with you through your caregiving season and your season of mourning, He has prepared you to help someone else. You are a part of God's plan because He knows you are capable; all HE asks is that you trust Him.

REFLECTIONS:

- Continue to journal your emotions. They will help you heal and help you when it's your turn to help someone else.

TRUSTING IN JESUS

"Do not let your heart be troubled. You have put your trust in God, put your trust in Me also." John14:1 (NLV)

Is your heart troubled by the loss of your loved one? Jesus is asking you to put your trust in Him; allowing Him to soothe your troubled heart and racing thoughts of despair and anxiety. Know that anxiety, despair, and lack of direction are not from God but from the enemy. It is his attempt to remove your focus from God and His plan for you. Putting your trust in Jesus means He will take care of YOU. The troubles will bow down to Him and His authority and the authority He has given You! However, you must choose to trust Him, choose to walk in accordance with His words, and choose to develop an ongoing growing relationship with HIM. You must choose!

Mourning is necessary because you will miss your loved one but mourning to the point of not being able to function is not what you, as a Christian, are! Walk with God and allow Him to love you through your season of mourning.

REFLECTIONS:

- Are you troubled? Why or why not?

ACTION STEPS:

- If you are troubled, list why, and pray over it; talk to the Lord about your anxieties. After praying over your list, throw it in the trash. This signifies that you have totally given your troubles to the Lord, except with confidence. He will see you through.

THE GOOD NEWS OF JESUS

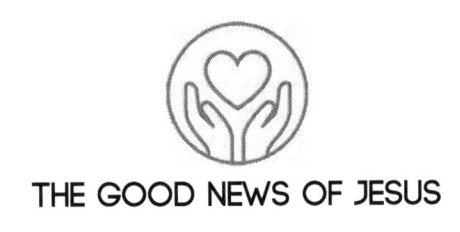

> "The Spirit of the Lord God is on me, because the Lord has chosen me to bring good news to poor people. He has sent me to heal those with a sad heart. He has sent me to tell those who are being held and those in prison that they can go free."
> Isaiah 61:1 (NLV)

Jesus! The hope of Glory is here! That is the good news that you have a Savior who loves and cares for you. He cared enough to die for you and cares for you now to be with you during your time of mourning. This was the first thing He declared publicly, and He did it because He knew you would need to be reminded. He came to heal your sad heart. Take comfort in this scripture today and your relationship with your Savior. Notice that His arrival marked the end of your captivity, from the captivity of sorrow and pain and the captivity of a loss of hope. Today remember what Jesus proclaims and then turn to His Spirit for comfort.

REFLECTIONS:

- Think of everything being in a relationship with Jesus means to you. Ponder your life if you were not in a relationship with Him.
- Talk with your heavenly Father (thank Him for Jesus and your relationship. Thank Him for not leaving you alone).

A GOD WHO CARES

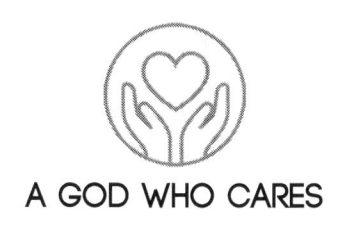

"Yet it was our weaknesses he carried; it was our sorrows that weighed him down. And we thought his troubles were a punishment from God, a punishment for his own sins!"
Isaiah 53:4 (NLT)

God cares for you. It was you He was thinking of as He went to the cross, and as He died on the cross, YOU were on His mind. He carried all the hurt, sorrow, and grief you are experiencing. This is important for you to remember because it reassures YOU that you are loved, and this feeling of sadness and sorrow will not overtake you nor hinder you from God's love. Allow His comfort to engulf you as you grieve for your loved one.

REFLECTIONS

- Take time to really think about what Jesus went through for YOU. Then thank Him and ask Him to help you through this time of mourning.

CELEBRATING YOUR LOVED ONE

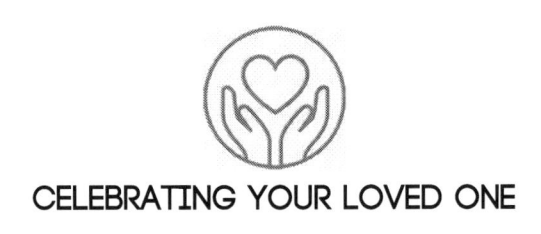

> "Ezra said to them, 'Go, eat and drink what you enjoy, and give some to him who has nothing ready. For this day is holy to our Lord. Do not be sad for the joy of the Lord is your strength.'"
> Nehemiah 8:10 (NLV)

As your caregiving journey ends, many emotions will flood your heart: loss, sadness, anger again, hopelessness, being numb, and despondence. However, as a child of the Most High God, you know that your loved one is now resting in the presence of their Savior. Allow this to comfort you and bring you out of the emotions listed above and instead allow you to feel joy, peace, and fullness. Fullness in knowing that you have completed this particular season God assigned you, peace in knowing your loved one is with Jesus, and joy resulting from the first two.

For the believer, the world expects you to mourn, and you will, but what you must also incorporate is CELEBRATING the LIFE of your loved one. Celebrate all they were and are to you and those they touched.

REFLECTIONS:

- Remember all the wonderful things that made your loved one so special.

PRAYER:

Talk to the Lord and ask Him to continue strengthening you as you transition out of this season.

A FINISHED RACE

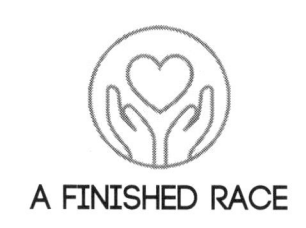

> "I have fought the good fight, I have finished the course, I have kept the faith; in the future there is laid up for me the crown of righteousness, which the Lord, the righteous Judge, will award to me on that day; and not only to me, but also to all who have loved His appearing." 2 Timothy 4:7-8 (NASB)

In grieving the loss of your loved one, don't forget to celebrate the race they have completed and won. God had a plan for them, and when His plan was completed, the Lord welcomed your loved one home. They are celebrating and have now joined that great cloud of witnesses referenced in Hebrews 12:1.

You also have a course or race that you must run, and this season of caring for your loved one is a segment you have now completed. Celebrate it. Hear God saying, "Well done, good and faithful servant." God is a righteous judge and will award you for your faithfulness. We are one body united in Christ for His purpose. Your loved one is now HOME.

REFLECTIONS:

- What does home mean to you?
- Do you know the race God has placed before you to run?
- Will you continue with the race?

PRAYER:

Dear Lord, thank You for the time You gave me with _____. I think it was too short because I didn't have enough time to love _____! Yet I know that I will see them again. I know You leaving me here means You still have something for me to do. I ask that You make it very clear and help me through this season of loss, remembering all the wonderful memories I made with _____, but that there are new memories to be made. I trust You, Lord, in Jesus' Name, Amen.

MY PRAYER FOR YOU

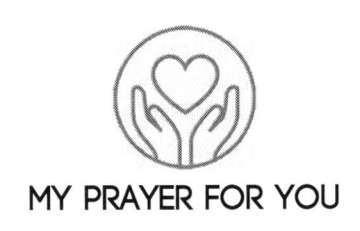

> "I pray that God, the source of hope, will fill you completely with joy and peace because you trust in him. Then you will overflow with confident hope through the power of the Holy Spirit."
> Romans 15:13 (NLT)

I pray that through this devotional, you have become more firm in your foundation and relationship with God and that you are completely filled with His joy and peace and your trust in Him. Please know that God loves you and that when it is your turn to enter into the Kingdom of Heaven, He will greet you with, "Well done."

MY PRAYER:

Lord, I thank You for my dear brother or sister. They have surrendered their lives to You and have obeyed Your call to caregiving. I thank You that they have grown closer to You through each step and have a more intimate relationship with You. Please help them know that You will continue to be with them and that You expect them to continue to walk closely with You. I ask that You protect them and cover them with Your mighty hand. LORD, bless and protect them; may You look upon them and smile and be gracious to them. I ask that You show favor to them and give them Your peace. In Jesus' Name, Amen.

REFLECTIONS
ACTION STEPS
PRAYERS

forWord BOOKS

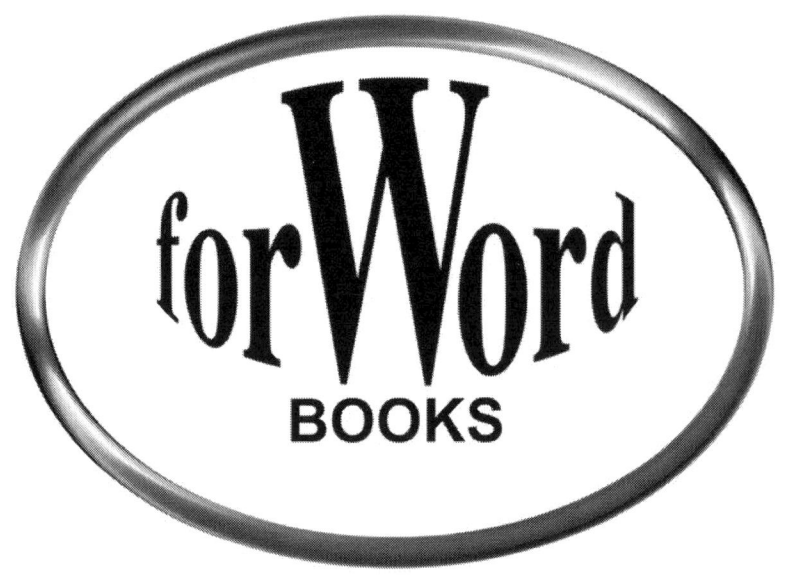

John 1:1 In the beginning was the Word...

CONTACT US VIA EMAIL AT FORWORDBOOKS@GMAIL.COM

Made in the USA
Las Vegas, NV
29 September 2023